No Gallbi Diet Cookbook

Start Your New Life Without a Gallbladder with 1800 Days of Simple and Delicious Recipes and a 45-Day Meal Plan to Optimize Digestion and Wellness

Nancy Walton

TABLE OF CONTENTS

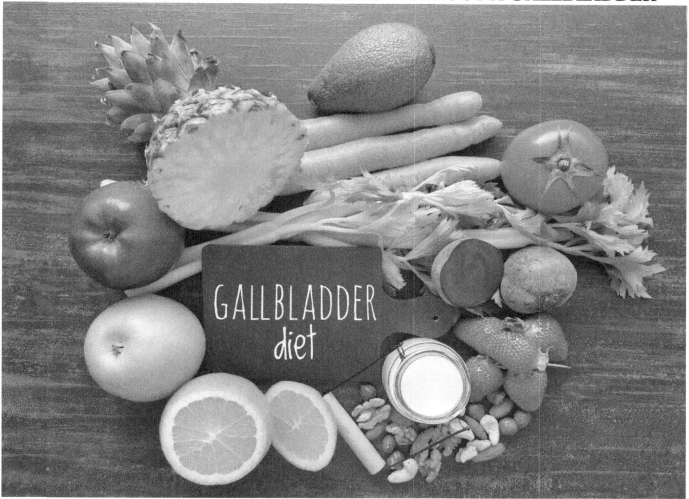

Welcome to the beginning of your journey to understanding life without a gallbladder. You've likely gone through the anxiety and relief that accompanies the decision to remove this small, yet significant organ. Now, as you navigate this new terrain, you might find yourself wondering how its absence will affect your daily life and health.

The loss of your gallbladder isn't just a surgical change but an invitation to reacquaint yourself with your body's needs. Think of your digestive system as a bustling city, with its highways, local traffic, and rules. Your gallbladder once acted as a traffic controller, managing the flow of bile into your intestines, crucial for digesting fats. Now, imagine that the traffic controller is on an indefinite leave. The bile still flows directly from your liver but in a steady, less regulated stream. This new rhythm might cause some initial disruptions perhaps bouts of indigestion or changes in your bowel movements.

This chapter is designed to offer you practical insights and empower you with knowledge about your body's new way of functioning. As challenging as it might seem initially, adapting to life without a gallbladder opens a door to a healthier, more attuned way of dining and living. It's about learning which foods invite comfort and health and those that might lead to discomfort. But it's more than just choosing the right ingredients; it's about embracing a new lifestyle that respects and supports your altered digestion.

In exploring these pages, you'll find the tools not only to manage but thrive in your post-gallbladder removal life. We'll discuss the common issues many face and provide effective strategies for dietary adjustments that fit smoothly into your life's puzzle. It's not merely about avoiding discomfort but enhancing your wellbeing through tailored nutritional choices, turning potential obstacles into stepping stones for greater health.

Here's to beginning this chapter with optimism and the commitment to learn, adapt, and flourish with a no gallbladder diet that supports and uplifts you every step of the way.

•1.1 THE GALLBLADDER'S ROLE IN DIGESTION: UNVEILING ITS FUNCTIONS AND IMPACT.

To truly appreciate the journey you are embarking on post-gallbladder removal, it's vital to first understand the role this small, pear-shaped organ played in your body. Nestled beneath your liver, the gallbladder was more than just a passive storage pouch for bile; it was an active, dynamic participant in your digestive process, particularly in the digestion of fats.

Bile, which is produced by the liver, serves as a detergent-like substance that aids in breaking down fats from the food you consume. It emulsifies fats, effectively turning large fat droplets into smaller ones—a process vital for the lipase enzymes to effectively do their job in breaking down dietary fats into fatty acids and glycerol, which your body can then use or store accordingly.

When you ate a meal that contained fats, a beautifully coordinated dance ensued. Your stomach would send a signal, and in response, your gallbladder would contract, squeezing concentrated bile through the bile ducts right into your small intestine. There, it worked its magic, making the fats easier to absorb and process. It's not just about aiding digestion; this process was crucial for absorbing fat-soluble vitamins (A, D, E, and K), supporting your immune system, and even helping to maintain your skin and eye health.

With the removal of your gallbladder, this process adjusts. Your liver continues to produce bile, but now it drips continuously into the small intestine, rather than being delivered in concentrated bursts. Without your gallbladder's regulation, the amount of bile available at any given time might not align perfectly with your dietary intake. This can lead to potential challenges, such as feelings of indigestion or a quicker transit of food through your colon, which may not allow enough time for these vital processes.

Navigating life post-gallbladder removal means recreating a balance in this new digestive landscape. It's empowering to consider that your body is remarkably adaptable. Although your digestive system operates differently now, you can adopt dietary habits that support this new mode. For instance, smaller, more frequent meals can prevent an overwhelming influx of fats that your system might struggle to process all at once. This not only minimizes discomfort but also optimizes the digestion and absorption of nutrients, aligning with your body's new method of processing dietary fats.

Moreover, the quality of fats you consume now holds a significant place in your diet. Emphasizing foods with healthy fats, such as avocados, nuts, and seeds, and using cooking oils like olive oil in moderation, can create an environment that eases your body's digestive process. These fats are not just easier on your digestion; they also contribute to overall health, offering essential fatty acids and helping to absorb those crucial vitamins your body needs.

Understanding these dynamics also sheds light on why particular symptoms might arise. For example, experiencing bloating or diarrhea after eating fatty meals isn't just a nuisance; it's a signal from your body that the balance isn't quite right. It invites an exploration into adjusting meal sizes, timing, and nutrient balance to better align with your current digestive capabilities.

This new understanding of your body's processes can offer a comforting sense of control and influence over your health. It supports not only the physical adaptation to living without a gallbladder but also engages you in an ongoing dialogue with your body, responding to its needs with thoughtful choices in your diet and lifestyle.

Living without a gallbladder isn't about facing a lifetime of dietary limitations or discomfort. Rather, it's about adapting and thriving within a new set of digestive dynamics. It is a profound journey of relearning and listening—tuning in to the signs your body gives and responding with care. This journey can deepen the connection to your body, enhancing your overall wellbeing and allowing you to live fully, even without a gallbladder.

Managing Fat Intake Your body's capacity to handle large amounts of fat at one sitting has diminished. You might find that foods which were once staples in your diet now trigger discomfort. This is your body's way of signaling its new limits. Emphasizing lean proteins, whole grains, and vegetables, while limiting high-fat items, can mitigate symptoms like diarrhea or cramping. Gradually reintroducing small amounts of healthy fats, such as those found in avocados or nuts, helps your body adapt without the harsh side effects.

Bile Acid Malabsorption In some cases, the continuous flow of bile can lead to an excess in the intestines, especially if it's not all needed for digestion. This surplus can irritate the lining of your intestines, leading to bile acid diarrhea. Here, a solution could include a bile acid binder, a medication that works by binding to the bile acids in the intestine and preventing them from causing diarrhea. It's a practical approach, but like any medication, it should be discussed and managed under the guidance of a healthcare professional.

Food Sensitivities Post-surgery, your tolerance to certain foods may change. Keeping a food diary can be an invaluable tool. By recording what you eat and any symptoms that follow, patterns can emerge that highlight specific food sensitivities. This ongoing record provides a clear guide to making informed adjustments that can alleviate symptoms and enhance your dietary satisfaction.

Nutrient Absorption With changes in your bile management, absorbing sufficient fat-soluble vitamins (A, D, E, K) can become a challenge. These nutrients are crucial for everything from vision to bone health. Supplements can bridge the gap, but they should be tailored to your specific needs and used under medical supervision. Ensuring that your meals are balanced and nutrient-dense also supports overall nutrient intake.

Emotional and Psychological Adjustments The physical adjustments are paralleled by psychological ones. Changes in your diet and lifestyle, coupled with managing symptoms, can evoke feelings of frustration or restriction. It's important to acknowledge these feelings; they are a valid part of your transition. Engaging with a supportive community, whether online or in person, can provide not only practical advice but also encouragement. Sharing experiences and solutions with others on similar journeys can reaffirm that you are not navigating these waters alone.

Long-term Management Strategies Looking beyond the initial adjustment phase, long-term management involves developing a deep understanding of your body's new rhythms and needs. Regular consultations with healthcare providers, such as a nutritionist or a gastroenterologist, will help fine-tune your diet and ensure that you are not only managing symptoms but thriving. Regular physical activity, tailored to your condition and fitness level, can also improve digestive efficiency and overall well-being.

Creating a New Normal Adapting to life without a gallbladder is not just about subtracting certain foods or grappling with discomfort but about creating a new normal—a lifestyle characterized by awareness, adjustment, and renewal. Each step you take to understand and adapt to your body's new way of functioning is a step towards reclaiming your quality of life and health. As daunting as these waters may seem initially, equipped with knowledge and the right strategies, you can steer through them towards a lifestyle that not only accommodates your post-gallbladder removal status but also enhances your overall health and well-being. Like any significant change, it offers an opportunity for renewal and growth. With each challenge managed, you'll gain not just comfort but also a deeper connection with and understanding of your body's new dynamics.

•1.3 Dietary Adaptation: Strategies for successful dietary transitions.

Embarking on a journey of dietary adaptation after gallbladder removal is like learning a new language. At first, it may seem daunting, navigating different sensations and reactions, but with dedication and the right strategies, you can fluently speak the language of your new digestive system, allowing for a seamless integration into your daily life.

Understanding Your New Digestive Dynamics Initially, the main goal post-surgery is to understand the new dynamics of your digestion. Without your gallbladder, your liver will deliver bile directly into your small intestine at a consistent but unregulated rate, which can lead to various digestive reactions when you consume fatty foods. To align you're eating habits with your body's changed capabilities, starting with a thorough observation period is essential. Take note of how different foods affect your body, which ones enhance your wellbeing, and which ones to avoid.

Gradual Integration A gradual approach helps ease your body into the changes. Start with a low-fat diet immediately after surgery to minimize stress on your digestive system. Slowly introduce different foods and monitor how your body responds. This slow and steady exploration allows your body to adapt without overwhelming it.

Moderation and Balance Balance is crucial. While your body may struggle with high-fat meals, it's critical to ensure you are still consuming enough healthy fats necessary for overall health. Incorporate small amounts of healthy fats gradually and consistently observe how your body manages these additions. This strategy helps in making adjustments that are both manageable and sustainable.

Meal Planning and Smaller Portions Meal planning can be a powerful tool in your new dietary regimen. Planning helps in spacing out meals to prevent overwhelming your system and ensuring you incorporate a variety of nutrients that support digestive health and overall wellness. Smaller, more frequent meals can also prevent the heavy influx of fats and promote easier digestion and nutrient absorption.

Listening to Your Body's Signals Your body has a unique way of communicating its needs and limits. It's important to become attuned to these signals. Symptoms such as bloating, gas, or diarrhea are not merely inconveniences but messages alerting you that adjustments are needed. This active listening leads to a deeper understanding and better management of your dietary needs.

Incorporating Digestive Aids Certain natural aids and supplements can assist in managing digestion and enhancing nutrient absorption. For instance, digestive enzymes can help in breaking down foods more efficiently, especially during the initial adjustment period. Similarly, soluble fiber can aid in regulating bowel movements and supporting a healthy digestive process. However, it is crucial to consult with a healthcare professional before introducing any supplements or significant changes to your diet.

Hydration and Its Role Hydration plays a critical role in your digestion. Water helps in the efficient flow of nutrients and the elimination of waste. It also aids in bile production and can dilute the bile, potentially reducing symptoms of discomfort. Ensuring adequate water intake is a simple yet effective strategy to support your digestive system.

Educational Resources and Support Arming yourself with knowledge is empowering. Understanding the physiological changes, nutritional needs, and potential complications post-gallbladder removal provides a foundation for making informed dietary choices. Additionally, seeking support from nutritionists who specialize in post-gallbladder removal diets can provide tailored advice and reassurance.

Embracing Change with a Positive Outlook Finally, the journey to adapting your diet post-gallbladder removal is not just about avoiding discomfort but about embracing a lifestyle that promotes optimal health and vitality. It's about seeing this change as an opportunity to enhance your life, discovering new foods and recipes that nourish and delight, and cultivating a positive relationship with food that respects your body's new way of functioning.

This approach to dietary adaptation is not merely about following a set of rules but about engaging in a dynamic process of learning, adjusting, and thriving. As you actively participate in this process, your confidence in managing your diet will grow, leading to improved health and a more joyful eating experience. Your diet, much like life, is a journey enriched not just by the foods you eat but by the greater understanding and connection you develop with your body.

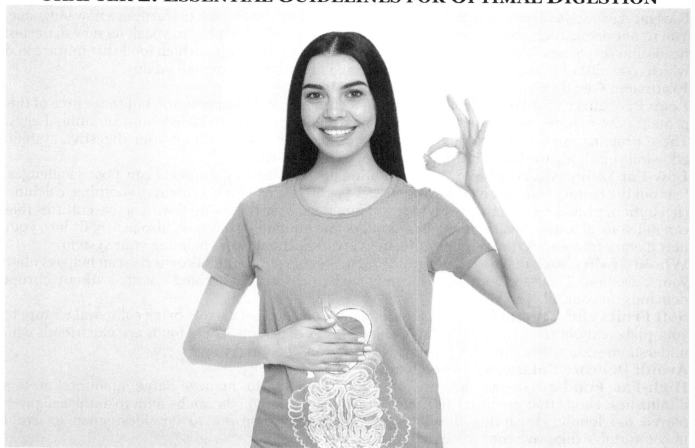

Embarking on a journey without a gallbladder can seem daunting, but with the right guidelines, it transforms into an opportunity to cultivate a more sensitive, attuned relationship with your body. Imagine your digestive system as a newly tuned instrument, and your diet as the music played upon it—when harmonized correctly, the melody of your daily life sings health and well-being.

Navigating this new terrain requires understanding which foods soothe and which provoke, a knowledge vital for anyone who has undergone gallbladder removal. It's not just about avoiding discomfort; it's about empowering yourself to make choices that enhance your digestion and contribute positively to your overall health.

Think of the times you might have felt bewildered in a bustling supermarket aisle, bombarded by an array of choices yet unsure of what's truly beneficial for your unique needs. Now, imagine yourself as an informed consumer, someone with insider knowledge about which foods to embrace lovingly and which to sidestep gracefully.

Here, in this chapter, we will delve into the essential dietary components to consider post-gallbladder removal. From understanding the pivotal role of fats and the types most conducive to your health, to recognizing how fiber can be your ally, albeit balanced and introduced thoughtfully. We'll explore how beautifully some foods can support the bile flow, aiding in the gentle digestion that your body now prefers.

Furthermore, the significance of structured meal patterns will not go unnoticed. Regular eating schedules do more than organize your day; they stabilize your digestive system's rhythm, helping to manage bile flow and reduce the chances of digestive distress.

Join me as we look beyond mere eating into constructing a lifestyle that supports optimal digestion through thoughtful choices—transforming challenges into a testament of resilience and health. Let's lay down the foundational knowledge that will not only alleviate apprehension but will enhance and nurture your life without a gallbladder.

•2.1 FOODS TO EMBRACE OR AVOID: COMPREHENSIVE LISTS AND EXPLANATIONS.

Navigating your dietary needs after gallbladder removal can be likened to learning a new language. You're not just eating; you're communicating with your body, learning to speak its new dialect of needs and responses. The nuances of this language involve discerning which foods to embrace and which to avoid, a vital skill for maintaining optimal digestion and overall vitality.

Embrace: Gentle Guides to Your Digestive Journey

Lean Proteins: Your body still needs protein for healing and maintenance, but the source of this protein now requires more consideration. Think tender poultry, flaky fish, and scrambled eggs. These proteins are not only easy to prepare but also put less strain on your digestive system, allowing your body to absorb nutrients without excessive stress.

Low-Fat Dairy Alternatives: While traditional high-fat dairy products can pose challenges, fear not the realm of alternatives. Low-fat Greek yogurt, for example, remains a soothing, calcium-rich option, providing the creamy texture you might miss, supplemented with active cultures that can aid your digestive health. Plant-based milks like almond or oat milk also gently fit into your new dietary framework, providing comforting flavors without overwhelming your system.

Whole Grains: Rich in fiber, whole grains such as oats, quinoa, and brown rice can help regulate your digestion. They are your slow-burning fuels, providing sustained energy without abrupt demands on your bile production.

Soft Fruits and Vegetables: Avocados, bananas, and cooked carrots bring color and texture to your plate without the harsh fibers that challenge your digestion. These foods are like friends who understand your needs and offer comfort without overwhelming you.

Avoid: Delicate Balances Not to Overwhelm

High-Fat Foods: Post-gallbladder, your body's ability to manage large amounts of fats diminishes. Foods that are heavy in butter, cream, and animal fats can be akin to a musical piece played too loudly, disrupting the harmony you seek. These are to be sidestepped to avoid uncomfortable digestive concerts of bloating and pain.

Fried and Processed Foods: Such items often contain hidden fats and oils that can sneak up on your digestive tract, causing flare-ups in what might otherwise be a smooth experience. Just as a jazz musician avoids discordant notes to keep the melody smooth, so should your diet avoid these disruptive elements.

Spicy and Acidic Foods: While they add zest and vibrancy to meals, overly spicy or acidic foods can provoke your digestive system in unwanted ways. Imagine these as the bold, high notes in music – thrilling yet potentially overpowering if your system isn't geared to handle them.

Cruciferous Vegetables: While incredibly healthy, vegetables like broccoli, cauliflower, and cabbages can cause gas and bloating when your gallbladder is absent. These might be considered the complex polyrhythms in the world of jazz—fascinating yet complex patterns that are challenging to digest in the literal sense.

Understanding the Symphony of Foods

Imagine each meal as a composition. The ingredients you choose contribute to either harmony or dissonance. Incorporating the right foods builds chords that resonate with health and balance; on the other hand, the wrong ones can cause a cacophony, disrupting the rhythmic flow of your digestion.

Mindfulness in eating transforms these choices into a daily practice of nurturing. With each meal, you're playing a chord that either supports your body's new way of functioning post-gallbladder or challenges it. It requires attention like tuning a violin, ensuring each string, each note, harmonizes perfectly into the melody you aim to achieve for your wellness.

Gradually, you begin to learn which foods sing in harmony with your body's needs and which clash. This knowledge becomes your guide, a trusted map as you navigate through the daily choices of nourishment.

In essence, the way forward isn't just about avoidance; it's about discovering new delights and revisiting old favorites in moderation and balance. Every bite is a note in your digestive symphony, and with careful composition, this symphony can be as vibrant and fulfilling as any feast enjoyed before your surgery. Together, through thoughtful choice and culinary creativity, resilience becomes not just a goal, but a delightful, daily reality.

•2.2 IMPORTANCE OF BALANCED NUTRITION: KEY NUTRIENTS AND THEIR BENEFITS.

Imagine standing in the middle of a lush garden, every plant representing a nutrient vital to your health, particularly after gallbladder removal. Understanding which plants to nurture and which are less essential is key to maintaining the garden of your body's wellbeing. Balanced nutrition isn't just about choosing the right foods; it's about fostering a deeper harmony within, ensuring each part of you thrives in the absence of your gallbladder.

After gallbladder surgery, your body undergoes significant adjustments, particularly in how it processes fats and absorbs nutrients. This transformation necessitates a meticulous reassessment of your nutritional intake to support optimal digestion and health. It's akin to recalibrating the instruments in an orchestra—every nutrient must play its part perfectly to produce a harmonious symphony of health.

Key Nutrients And Their Symphony of Benefits

Proteins: Like the robust beats of a drum, proteins are foundational for healing and repairing tissues post-surgery. Lean proteins such as chicken, turkey, fish, and legumes, provide the necessary amplitudes without overwhelming your system. They help stitch and strengthen the very fabric of your bodily tissues, promoting a recovery that is both resilient and refining.

Fats: Often misunderstood, especially post-gallbladder, fats remain an essential part of your nutrition. However, the key lies in choosing fats that are easier on your system—those that do not obligate your liver to work overtime. Think of monounsaturated and polyunsaturated fats, like those from avocados, nuts, and seeds, as the gentle strums of a harp, enriching the melody without drowning it.

Carbohydrates: Carbohydrates are the body's primary energy source, fueling your cells like wind powering sails. Opt for complex carbs from whole grains, vegetables, and fruits, which release energy steadily, keeping your digestive system balanced and active without abrupt spikes or drops in blood sugar. These are the sustaining rhythms that keep the body's rhythms regular and reliable.

Fibers: With the gallbladder gone, fibers take on an even more poignant role. Soluble fiber, found in foods like oats, apples, and carrots, helps to regulate digestion and assist in the smooth passage of food through your intestines. Think of them as the conductors of your gastrointestinal orchestra, maintaining tempo and flow within the digestive tract.

Vitamins and Minerals: Post-gallbladder, your body's ability to absorb certain vitamins and minerals, especially fat-soluble ones such as Vitamins A, D, E, and K, is reduced. It becomes crucial to incorporate foods rich in these nutrients or consider supplementation under medical guidance. These nutrients are like the vibrant bursts of a trumpet's call in an orchestra, essential not in quantity but in their power to invigorate and protect.

Water and Fluids: Beyond nutrition, hydration plays a critical role in maintaining digestive health. Water is the lifeblood of your body's landscape, ensuring nutrients flow where needed and cleansing systems of waste. Hydration in your diet can be likened to the acoustic resonance in a musical hall, necessary for the clarity and quality of the notes played by the orchestra.

Fine-Tuning Your Nutritional Orchestra

Balanced nutrition, especially in the absence of your gallbladder, is less about adhering to strict diets and more about listening—truly listening—to your body's responses. It's not just about eating healthily but about eating intelligently. Each meal, each nutrient, resonates differently within your body. By attuning yourself to these responses, you can orchestrate a diet that not only respects but enhances your new digestive landscape.

This tuning involves timing your meals to sync with your digest's natural rhythms, learning to pair nutrients for maximum absorption, and understanding portions to optimize digestive comfort.

Balanced nutrition becomes your lifelong commitment, a commitment to nourishing your body with every nourishing bite.

In this music of meals, each note is essential, each pause meaningful. As you harmonize your diet to fit your body's post-surgical needs, you not only ease the physical transitions but also support your broader health goals. From stronger immunity and improved tissue healing to sustained energy levels and mood stabilization, the benefits extend far beyond digestion.

Embrace this journey of relearning and recalibration. Let the knowledge of balanced nutrition be your guide, and the practice of mindful eating your pathway to a vibrant, harmonious life. With each mindful choice, you are composing your health's masterpiece, resonant with the beauty and balance of well-being.

•2.3 Digestive Health Tips: Practical advice for everyday wellness.

Visualize yourself embarking on a serene morning walk, where each step represents a day in your journey towards digestive health post-gallbladder removal. Just as walking steadily and rhythmically can enhance your physical wellness, integrating specific, practical habits into your daily routine can significantly boost your digestive health. Each habit, simple yet powerful, acts as a stepping stone towards a smoother digestive process and an enriched life.

Embracing Regularity and Mindfulness

Establishing a routine can be as beneficial for your digestive system as it is for your mental state. Regular meal times not only condition your body to expect and efficiently handle food intake, but they also maintain a steady flow of bile, reducing the potential for it to sit and concentrate, which can lead to discomfort. Imagine this regularity as a gentle, rhythmic dance that keeps your digestive system in grace and harmony.

Mindfulness while eating goes beyond merely chewing slowly. It involves engaging all your senses, appreciating the colors, textures, and flavors of your food. This practice helps you recognize satiety cues, preventing overeating, which can be particularly troublesome when your gallbladder is absent. Consider each meal an opportunity to connect with your food, allowing full mental participation to guide your physical intake.

Simplifying Meals

In the post-gallbladder removal life, simpler meals often equate to happier digestion. Complex meals with excessive ingredients can be harder to digest. Think of your meal as a piece of music— the more instruments involved, the greater the complexity; similarly, a dish with fewer components is easier for your body to orchestrate. Lean proteins, steamed vegetables, and easy-to-digest grains form a trio that can perform beautifully together without overwhelming your system.

Hydration: The Unsung Hero

Hydration plays an understated yet critical role in maintaining digestive health. Water aids in the seamless flow of nutrients and prevents bile from becoming too concentrated, which is crucial when you're managing without a gallbladder. Integrating hydration into your daily life doesn't just mean drinking water—it could involve incorporating hydrating foods like cucumbers, zucchini, and watermelon, which can add variety and extra nutrients to your hydration efforts.

Gentle Movement

Gentle, regular physical activity such as walking, yoga, or light stretching can improve gut motility and aid in the effective movement of food through your digestive tract. Consider physical activity as the tempo of your digestive melody, with gentle movements setting a baseline rhythm that keeps everything moving along harmoniously.

Stress Management

Stress undeniably affects digestion. The gut is often referred to as the "second brain" because of the extensive network of neurons lining the gastrointestinal tract. Stress management techniques such as deep breathing exercises, mindfulness meditation, or engaging in hobbies can help soothe your nervous system and, in turn, calm your digestive system. Managing stress is akin to tuning an instrument, ensuring it produces a sound that is pleasant and harmonious, rather than jarring and disruptive.

Smart Snacking

While large meals can burden your digestive system, smart snacking can keep your energy levels steady without overtaxing your digestion. Snacks rich in fiber, protein, and healthy fats can provide sustained energy and aid in digestion. Almonds, carrots with hummus, or an apple with peanut butter are examples of snacks that harmonize well with your dietary needs, providing nourishment without the digestive drama.

Listening to Your Body

Above all, listening attentively to your body remains your most reliable guide. Each person's reaction to having no gallbladder is unique, and what works for one might not work for another. Tracking your meals and their effects, noting what soothes and what irritates, can provide you personalized insights into your optimal dietary harmony.

Imagine these practices not just as isolated actions but as components of a comprehensive melody that you are composing day by day. Together, they form a lifestyle symphony that promotes not only digestive health but also a holistic sense of well-being.

By adopting these practices, you are not merely adjusting to life without a gallbladder; you are embracing a lifestyle that places premium care on your digestive system, learning to manage it with grace and efficiency. Through these tips, you find not just recovery but a renewed rhythm of life that resonates with health and vitality. Each day unfolds as a continuing exploration of the delicate balance that defines your digestive wellness.

CHAPTER 3: BREAKFAST RECIPES - STARTING YOUR DAY RIGHT

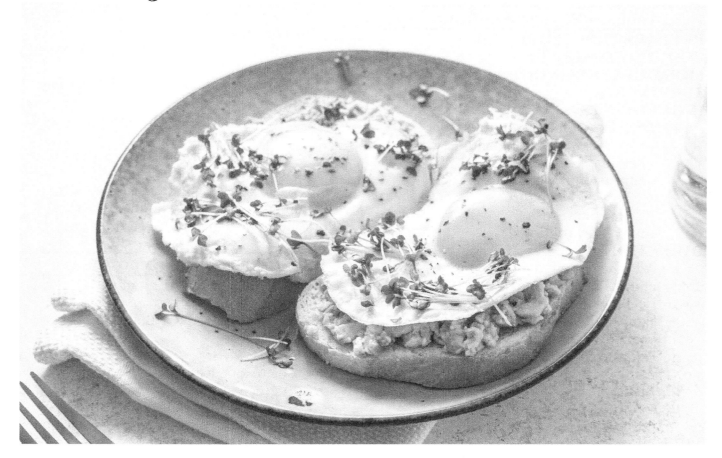

Imagine waking up to the gentle hum of the morning, the sun casting a golden hue across the sky. The day is fresh, brimming with possibilities, and what better way to embrace its potential than with a nourishing breakfast? Breakfast, often heralded as the most important meal of the day, serves as the foundation for our daily endeavors. It's a moment of tranquility, a pause before the whirlwind of daily tasks, where we can nurture our bodies and minds with wholesome food.

As the world rushes around us, the simplicity of a well-prepared breakfast offers a moment of solace. It's a ritual that grounds us, connecting the past and the future with the present. Whether it's the comforting aroma of freshly brewed coffee, the vibrant colors of a fruit-laden smoothie, or the warmth of a bowl of oats, breakfast holds the power to transform our mornings from mundane to magical.

In this chapter, we'll explore a variety of breakfast recipes designed to cater to diverse tastes and dietary needs. From energizing smoothies that blend the goodness of fruits and vegetables into a refreshing start, to hearty breakfast bowls that combine grains, proteins, and fresh produce into a meal that fuels you through the morning. We'll delve into the simplicity of egg dishes, showcasing how this versatile ingredient can be the star of a satisfying breakfast with minimal effort.

Each recipe is crafted with care, emphasizing the balance between taste and nutrition. The goal is to inspire you to create breakfasts that are not only delicious but also nourishing, setting a positive tone for the rest of the day. As you navigate through these recipes, you'll find that breakfast can be more than just a routine it can be a celebration of the new day, a reason to rise and shine with enthusiasm.

So, let's embark on this culinary journey together. Let's rediscover the joy of breakfast, one recipe at a time, and make each morning a testament to the power of good food and good beginnings.

TROPICAL SUNRISE SMOOTHIE

PREPARATION TIME: 10 min
COOKING TIME: N/A
MODE OF COOKING: Blending
SERVINGS: 2
INGREDIENTS:
- 1 cup frozen mango chunks
- 1 cup frozen pineapple chunks
- 1 banana
- 1 cup coconut water
- 1/2 cup Greek yogurt
- 1 Tbsp chia seeds
- 1 tsp honey (optional)

DIRECTIONS:
1. Add the frozen mango and pineapple chunks to the blender.
2. Peel and add the banana.
3. Pour in the coconut water and Greek yogurt.
4. Add the chia seeds and honey, if using.
5. Blend until smooth and creamy.
6. Pour into glasses and serve immediately.

TIPS:
- For a thicker smoothie, add a handful of ice cubes.
- Substitute coconut water with almond milk for a creamier texture.

N.V.: Calories: 210, Fat: 3.5g, Carbs: 45g, Protein: 7g, Sugar: 34g, Sodium: 90 mg, Potassium: 600 mg, Cholesterol: 0 mg

BERRY BLAST SMOOTHIE

PREPARATION TIME: 5 min
COOKING TIME: N/A
MODE OF COOKING: Blending
SERVINGS: 2
INGREDIENTS:
- 1 cup mixed berries (strawberries, blueberries, raspberries)
- 1 banana
- 1 cup spinach leaves
- 1 cup unsweetened almond milk
- 1 Tbsp flax seeds
- 1 tsp vanilla extract

DIRECTIONS:
1. Add the mixed berries and banana to the blender.
2. Add the spinach leaves.
3. Pour in the almond milk.
4. Add the flax seeds and vanilla extract.
5. Blend until smooth.
6. Serve immediately in chilled glasses.

TIPS:
- Use frozen berries for a colder, thicker smoothie.
- Add a scoop of protein powder for an extra protein boost.

N.V.: Calories: 180, Fat: 4g, Carbs: 38g, Protein: 4g, Sugar: 24g, Sodium: 130 mg, Potassium: 500 mg, Cholesterol: 0 mg

GREEN DETOX SMOOTHIE

PREPARATION TIME: 5 min
COOKING TIME: N/A
MODE OF COOKING: Blending
SERVINGS: 2
INGREDIENTS:
- 1 cup kale leaves
- 1 green apple, cored and chopped
- 1/2 cucumber, sliced
- 1/2 lemon, juiced
- 1 cup coconut water
- 1 Tbsp fresh ginger, grated

DIRECTIONS:
1. Add the kale leaves to the blender.
2. Add the chopped green apple and sliced cucumber.
3. Squeeze in the lemon juice.
4. Pour in the coconut water.
5. Add the grated ginger.
6. Blend until smooth.
7. Serve in tall glasses.

TIPS:
- Add a few ice cubes to chill the smoothie.
- Substitute coconut water with regular water for a less sweet option.

N.V.: Calories: 90, Fat: 0.5g, Carbs: 23g, Protein: 2g, Sugar: 14g, Sodium: 40 mg, Potassium: 450 mg, Cholesterol: 0 mg

CREAMY AVOCADO SMOOTHIE

PREPARATION TIME: 5 min
COOKING TIME: N/A
MODE OF COOKING: Blending
SERVINGS: 2
INGREDIENTS:

- 1 ripe avocado
- 1 banana
- 1 cup spinach leaves
- 1 cup unsweetened almond milk
- 1 Tbsp honey
- 1/2 tsp cinnamon

DIRECTIONS:

1. Scoop out the avocado and add to the blender.
2. Add the banana and spinach leaves.
3. Pour in the almond milk.
4. Add the honey and cinnamon.
5. Blend until smooth and creamy.
6. Pour into glasses and serve.

TIPS:

- Add a handful of ice cubes for a chilled smoothie.
- Use a high-powered blender for the best consistency.

N.V.: Calories: 220, Fat: 12g, Carbs: 28g, Protein: 3g, Sugar: 14g, Sodium: 60 mg, Potassium: 650 mg, Cholesterol: 0 mg

PROTEIN POWER SMOOTHIE

PREPARATION TIME: 5 min
COOKING TIME: N/A
MODE OF COOKING: Blending
SERVINGS: 2
INGREDIENTS:

- 1 cup unsweetened almond milk
- 1 banana
- 1 scoop vanilla protein powder
- 1 Tbsp almond butter
- 1 Tbsp cocoa powder
- 1/2 tsp cinnamon
- 1 Tbsp chia seeds

DIRECTIONS:

1. Pour the almond milk into the blender.
2. Add the banana and protein powder.
3. Add the almond butter, cocoa powder, cinnamon, and chia seeds.
4. Blend until smooth.
5. Serve immediately in protein shaker bottles or glasses.

TIPS:

- For a thicker smoothie, add a handful of ice cubes.
- Use peanut butter instead of almond butter for a different flavor profile.

N.V.: Calories: 290, Fat: 12g, Carbs: 30g, Protein: 18g, Sugar: 14g, Sodium: 200 mg, Potassium: 500 mg, Cholesterol: 0 mg

3.2 NUTRIENT-PACKED BREAKFAST BOWLS: IDEAS FOR A WHOLESOME MORNING MEAL.

QUINOA AND BERRY BREAKFAST BOWL

PREPARATION TIME: 10 min
COOKING TIME: 15 min
MODE OF COOKING: Stovetop
SERVINGS: 2
INGREDIENTS:

- 1 cup quinoa, rinsed
- 2 cups water
- 1/2 cup blueberries
- 1/2 cup strawberries, sliced
- 1 banana, sliced
- 1/4 cup almonds, sliced
- 1 Tbsp chia seeds
- 1/4 cup Greek yogurt
- 1 Tbsp honey
- 1/2 tsp cinnamon

DIRECTIONS:

1. In a medium saucepan, bring the quinoa and water to a boil.
2. Reduce heat to low, cover, and simmer for about 15 minutes or until quinoa is tender and water is absorbed.
3. Remove from heat and let it sit for 5 minutes, then fluff with a fork.
4. Divide the quinoa into two bowls.
5. Top each bowl with blueberries, strawberries, banana slices, almonds, and chia seeds.
6. Add a dollop of Greek yogurt to each bowl.
7. Drizzle with honey and sprinkle with cinnamon.
8. Serve immediately.

TIPS:

- Substitute Greek yogurt with coconut yogurt for a dairy-free option.
- Add a handful of spinach to the quinoa while cooking for extra nutrients.

N.V.: Calories: 350, Fat: 12g, Carbs: 55g, Protein: 12g, Sugar: 20g, Sodium: 40 mg, Potassium: 700 mg, Cholesterol: 0 mg

SAVORY AVOCADO AND EGG BREAKFAST BOWL

PREPARATION TIME: 10 min
COOKING TIME: 10 min
MODE OF COOKING: Stovetop
SERVINGS: 2
INGREDIENTS:

- 1 cup cooked brown rice
- 2 eggs
- 1 avocado, sliced
- 1/2 cup cherry tomatoes, halved
- 1/4 cup black beans, rinsed and drained
- 1 Tbsp olive oil
- 1 Tbsp lime juice
- 1/4 cup cilantro, chopped
- Salt and pepper to taste

DIRECTIONS:

1. Cook the brown rice according to package instructions.
2. In a small skillet, heat the olive oil over medium heat.
3. Crack the eggs into the skillet and cook until whites are set but yolks are still runny, about 3-4 minutes.
4. Divide the cooked rice into two bowls.
5. Top each bowl with an egg, avocado slices, cherry tomatoes, and black beans.
6. Drizzle with lime juice and sprinkle with cilantro, salt, and pepper.
7. Serve immediately.

TIPS:

- Add a dash of hot sauce for a spicy kick.
- Substitute brown rice with quinoa or farro for variety.

N.V.: Calories: 400, Fat: 22g, Carbs: 40g, Protein: 15g, Sugar: 3g, Sodium: 200 mg, Potassium: 700 mg, Cholesterol: 185 mg

PEANUT BUTTER BANANA OATMEAL BOWL

PREPARATION TIME: 5 min
COOKING TIME: 5 min
MODE OF COOKING: Stovetop
SERVINGS: 2
INGREDIENTS:

- 1 cup rolled oats
- 2 cups almond milk
- 1 banana, sliced
- 2 Tbsp peanut butter
- 1 Tbsp flax seeds
- 1 Tbsp honey
- 1/2 tsp cinnamon
- 1/4 cup walnuts, chopped

DIRECTIONS:

1. In a medium saucepan, combine the rolled oats and almond milk.
2. Bring to a boil over medium heat, then reduce to a simmer.
3. Cook, stirring occasionally, until oats are tender and the mixture is creamy, about 5 minutes.
4. Divide the oatmeal into two bowls.
5. Top each bowl with banana slices, peanut butter, flax seeds, honey, cinnamon, and chopped walnuts.
6. Serve immediately.

TIPS:

- Use steel-cut oats for a chewier texture.
- Add a splash of vanilla extract for extra flavor.

N.V.: Calories: 380, Fat: 16g, Carbs: 54g, Protein: 10g, Sugar: 18g, Sodium: 150 mg, Potassium: 500 mg, Cholesterol: 0 mg

TROPICAL ACAI BREAKFAST BOWL

PREPARATION TIME: 10 min
COOKING TIME: N/A
MODE OF COOKING: Blending
SERVINGS: 2
INGREDIENTS:

- 1 acai smoothie pack, frozen
- 1 banana
- 1/2 cup pineapple chunks
- 1/2 cup mango chunks
- 1/2 cup coconut water
- 1/4 cup granola
- 1/4 cup shredded coconut
- 1 Tbsp chia seeds
- 1 Tbsp honey

DIRECTIONS:

1. In a blender, combine the acai pack, banana, pineapple chunks, mango chunks, and coconut water.
2. Blend until smooth and thick.
3. Divide the mixture into two bowls.
4. Top each bowl with granola, shredded coconut, chia seeds, and a drizzle of honey.
5. Serve immediately.

TIPS:

- Use frozen fruit for a thicker texture.
- Add a handful of spinach for extra nutrients.

N.V.: Calories: 320, Fat: 10g, Carbs: 55g, Protein: 5g, Sugar: 32g, Sodium: 35 mg, Potassium: 700 mg, Cholesterol: 0 mg

SWEET POTATO AND SPINACH BREAKFAST BOWL

PREPARATION TIME: 10 min
COOKING TIME: 20 min
MODE OF COOKING: Stovetop
SERVINGS: 2
INGREDIENTS:

- 1 large sweet potato, peeled and diced
- 1 cup spinach leaves
- 1/2 avocado, sliced
- 2 eggs
- 1 Tbsp olive oil
- 1/4 tsp paprika
- Salt and pepper to taste

DIRECTIONS:

1. In a medium saucepan, bring water to a boil and add the diced sweet potato.
2. Cook for 10-12 minutes until tender, then drain.
3. In a skillet, heat olive oil over medium heat.
4. Add the cooked sweet potato and spinach leaves to the skillet.
5. Cook until the spinach is wilted, about 3-4 minutes.
6. Season with paprika, salt, and pepper.
7. In another small skillet, cook the eggs to your liking (fried, scrambled, or poached).
8. Divide the sweet potato and spinach mixture into two bowls.
9. Top each bowl with an egg and avocado slices.
10. Serve immediately.

TIPS:

- Add a squeeze of lemon juice for a fresh flavor.
- Substitute sweet potato with butternut squash for a different taste.

N.V.: Calories: 350, Fat: 18g, Carbs: 35g, Protein: 10g, Sugar: 8g, Sodium: 150 mg, Potassium: 800 mg, Cholesterol: 185 mg

CLASSIC SCRAMBLED EGGS

PREPARATION TIME: 5 min
COOKING TIME: 5 min
MODE OF COOKING: Stovetop
SERVINGS: 2
INGREDIENTS:

- 4 large eggs
- 1/4 cup milk (optional)
- 1 Tbsp butter
- Salt and pepper to taste
- 1/4 cup chives, chopped (optional)

DIRECTIONS:

1. In a bowl, whisk together the eggs, milk (if using), salt, and pepper until well combined.
2. Heat a non-stick skillet over medium heat and add the butter.
3. Once the butter is melted, pour in the egg mixture.
4. Let the eggs sit for a few seconds, then gently stir with a spatula, pushing from the edges to the center.
5. Continue to cook until eggs are set but still slightly creamy, about 2-3 minutes.
6. Remove from heat and sprinkle with chopped chives, if desired.
7. Serve immediately.

TIPS:

- Use a low heat setting to avoid overcooking.
- Add a splash of cream for extra richness.

N.V.: Calories: 210, Fat: 16g, Carbs: 2g, Protein: 14g, Sugar: 1g, Sodium: 170 mg, Potassium: 150 mg, Cholesterol: 380 mg

SPINACH AND FETA OMELET

PREPARATION TIME: 5 min
COOKING TIME: 5 min
MODE OF COOKING: Stovetop
SERVINGS: 2
INGREDIENTS:

- 4 large eggs
- 1/4 cup milk
- 1 cup fresh spinach, chopped
- 1/4 cup feta cheese, crumbled
- 1 Tbsp olive oil
- Salt and pepper to taste

DIRECTIONS:

1. In a bowl, whisk together the eggs, milk, salt, and pepper.
2. Heat the olive oil in a non-stick skillet over medium heat.
3. Add the chopped spinach and sauté until wilted, about 1 minute.
4. Pour the egg mixture over the spinach and cook until the edges begin to set, about 1-2 minutes.
5. Sprinkle the feta cheese over half of the omelet.
6. Fold the omelet in half and cook for another 1-2 minutes until fully set.
7. Serve immediately.

TIPS:

- Use baby spinach for a milder flavor.
- Add a pinch of nutmeg to enhance the spinach's taste.

N.V.: Calories: 250, Fat: 19g, Carbs: 4g, Protein: 17g, Sugar: 2g, Sodium: 350 mg, Potassium: 300 mg, Cholesterol: 380 mg

VEGGIE-PACKED EGG MUFFINS

PREPARATION TIME: 10 min
COOKING TIME: 20 min
MODE OF COOKING: Baking
SERVINGS: 4
INGREDIENTS:

- 6 large eggs
- 1/4 cup milk
- 1/2 cup bell peppers, diced
- 1/2 cup zucchini, diced
- 1/4 cup red onion, diced
- 1/4 cup cheddar cheese, shredded
- Salt and pepper to taste
- 1 Tbsp olive oil

DIRECTIONS:

1. Preheat oven to 375°F (190°C). Grease a muffin tin with olive oil.
2. In a bowl, whisk together the eggs, milk, salt, and pepper.
3. Divide the bell peppers, zucchini, and red onion evenly among the muffin cups.
4. Pour the egg mixture into each cup, filling them about 3/4 full.
5. Sprinkle shredded cheddar cheese on top of each muffin.

6. Bake for 20 minutes or until the egg muffins are set and lightly golden.
7. Allow to cool slightly before removing from the muffin tin.
8. Serve warm or at room temperature.

TIPS:
- Store leftovers in the refrigerator for up to 3 days.
- Customize with your favorite veggies or add cooked bacon or sausage.

N.V.: Calories: 150, Fat: 10g, Carbs: 4g, Protein: 11g, Sugar: 2g, Sodium: 250 mg, Potassium: 200 mg, Cholesterol: 280 mg

AVOCADO TOAST WITH POACHED EGGS

PREPARATION TIME: 10 min
COOKING TIME: 5 min
MODE OF COOKING: Stovetop
SERVINGS: 2
INGREDIENTS:
- 2 large eggs
- 2 slices whole grain bread
- 1 avocado, mashed
- 1 Tbsp lemon juice
- Salt and pepper to taste
- 1 Tbsp white vinegar
- 1/4 cup cherry tomatoes, halved (optional)

DIRECTIONS:
1. In a small bowl, mix the mashed avocado with lemon juice, salt, and pepper.
2. Toast the slices of whole grain bread to your liking.
3. Bring a pot of water to a gentle simmer and add the vinegar.
4. Crack the eggs into separate small bowls or cups.
5. Create a gentle whirlpool in the pot and carefully slide each egg into the water.
6. Poach the eggs for 3-4 minutes until whites are set but yolks are still runny.
7. Spread the avocado mixture evenly on each toast slice.
8. Top each with a poached egg and cherry tomato halves, if using.
9. Serve immediately.

TIPS:
- Use a ripe avocado for the best texture.
- Sprinkle with red pepper flakes for a bit of heat.

N.V.: Calories: 290, Fat: 20g, Carbs: 22g, Protein: 10g, Sugar: 2g, Sodium: 250 mg, Potassium: 600 mg, Cholesterol: 185 mg

MEDITERRANEAN EGG SKILLET

PREPARATION TIME: 10 min
COOKING TIME: 15 min
MODE OF COOKING: Stovetop
SERVINGS: 2
INGREDIENTS:
- 4 large eggs
- 1/4 cup feta cheese, crumbled
- 1 cup cherry tomatoes, halved
- 1/2 cup baby spinach
- 1/4 cup red onion, diced
- 2 Tbsp olive oil
- Salt and pepper to taste
- 1/4 tsp oregano
- 1/4 tsp paprika

DIRECTIONS:
1. Heat olive oil in a large skillet over medium heat.
2. Add the red onion and cook until softened, about 3 minutes.
3. Add the cherry tomatoes and cook until they begin to soften, about 2 minutes.
4. Stir in the baby spinach and cook until wilted, about 1 minute.
5. Create four small wells in the vegetable mixture and crack an egg into each well.
6. Sprinkle with salt, pepper, oregano, and paprika.
7. Cover the skillet and cook until eggs are set to your liking, about 5-7 minutes.
8. Sprinkle with crumbled feta cheese.
9. Serve directly from the skillet.

TIPS:
- Add olives for an extra Mediterranean touch.
- Serve with warm pita bread for a complete meal.

N.V.: Calories: 320, Fat: 24g, Carbs: 10g, Protein: 15g, Sugar: 4g, Sodium: 400 mg, Potassium: 500 mg, Cholesterol: 380 mg

CHAPTER 4: LUNCH RECIPES - MIDDAY NOURISHMENT

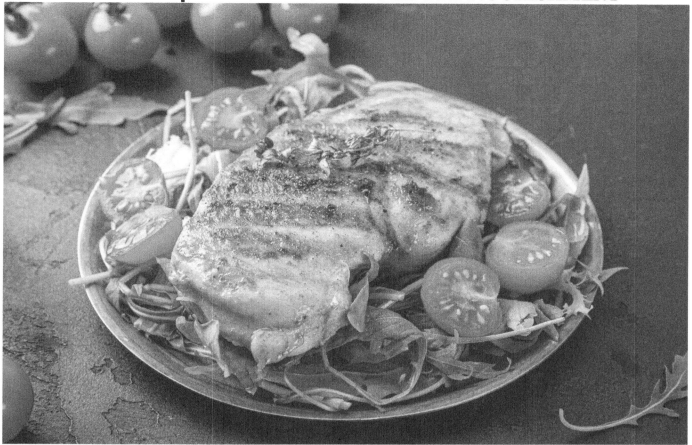

As the morning begins to wane and the sun reaches its zenith, our bodies and minds call for a pause a time to rejuvenate and replenish our energy with a wholesome midday meal. Lunch is more than just a break in the day; it is a vital moment of nourishment that bridges the morning's activities with the afternoon's demands. In the hustle of our daily routines, lunch often becomes a hurried affair, but it holds the potential to be a delightful and fulfilling experience.

Imagine the allure of a beautifully composed salad, crisp and fresh, drizzled with a tangy vinaigrette. Or picture the comforting embrace of a warm soup, its aromas filling the kitchen, promising comfort and satisfaction with every spoonful. Lunch can be a culinary adventure, a chance to explore flavors and ingredients that invigorate the senses and provide the sustenance we need to power through the rest of the day.

In this chapter, we dive into the world of lunch recipes crafted to nourish and delight. Each dish is designed to be as nutritious as it is flavorful, ensuring that your midday meal is a highlight rather than an afterthought. From vibrant salads bursting with fresh vegetables and lean proteins to hearty sandwiches that balance taste and texture, these recipes offer a variety of options to suit different preferences and dietary needs.

We'll also explore soothing soups and broths that are not only gentle on the digestive system but also rich in nutrients, providing a comforting break in the day. And for those moments when simplicity is key, you'll find easy-to-prepare meals that don't compromise on taste or nourishment. As you journey through these recipes, you'll discover that lunch can be an opportunity to recharge, a moment of mindfulness that sets the tone for a productive and enjoyable afternoon. Whether you are packing a meal for the office, enjoying a leisurely lunch at home, or sharing a meal with friends, these recipes aim to inspire and empower you to make the most of your midday nourishment.

So, let's embrace the possibilities of lunch, transforming it from a mere routine into a celebration of food, health, and well-being. Together, we'll explore the delicious potential that lies within each midday meal, ensuring that every bite contributes to our overall vitality and happiness.

•4.1 HEALTHY AND HEARTY SALADS: RECIPES FOR LIGHT, NUTRITIOUS MEALS.

QUINOA AND KALE SALAD

PREPARATION TIME: 15 min
COOKING TIME: 15 min
MODE OF COOKING: Stovetop
SERVINGS: 4
INGREDIENTS:
- 1 cup quinoa, rinsed
- 2 cups water
- 4 cups kale, chopped
- 1 cup cherry tomatoes, halved
- 1/2 cup cucumber, diced
- 1/4 cup red onion, thinly sliced
- 1/4 cup feta cheese, crumbled
- 1/4 cup almonds, sliced
- 1/4 cup olive oil
- 2 Tbsp lemon juice
- 1 tsp honey
- Salt and pepper to taste

DIRECTIONS:
1. In a medium saucepan, bring quinoa and water to a boil.
2. Reduce heat to low, cover, and simmer for 15 minutes or until quinoa is tender and water is absorbed.
3. Remove from heat and let sit for 5 minutes, then fluff with a fork.
4. In a large bowl, combine chopped kale, cherry tomatoes, cucumber, red onion, feta cheese, and almonds.
5. Add the cooked quinoa to the bowl and toss to combine.
6. In a small bowl, whisk together olive oil, lemon juice, honey, salt, and pepper.
7. Pour the dressing over the salad and toss to coat evenly.
8. Serve immediately or refrigerate until ready to serve.

TIPS:
- Massage the kale with a little olive oil and salt to soften it.
- Add avocado slices for extra creaminess.

N.V.: Calories: 320, Fat: 18g, Carbs: 32g, Protein: 9g, Sugar: 6g, Sodium: 180 mg, Potassium: 600 mg, Cholesterol: 15 mg

CHICKPEA AND AVOCADO SALAD

PREPARATION TIME: 10 min
COOKING TIME: N/A
MODE OF COOKING: N/A
SERVINGS: 4
INGREDIENTS:
- 2 cups chickpeas, cooked or canned (rinsed and drained)
- 1 avocado, diced
- 1 cup cherry tomatoes, halved
- 1/2 cup red bell pepper, diced
- 1/4 cup red onion, diced
- 1/4 cup cilantro, chopped
- 2 Tbsp olive oil
- 1 Tbsp lime juice
- 1 tsp cumin
- Salt and pepper to taste

DIRECTIONS:
1. In a large bowl, combine chickpeas, avocado, cherry tomatoes, red bell pepper, red onion, and cilantro.
2. In a small bowl, whisk together olive oil, lime juice, cumin, salt, and pepper.
3. Pour the dressing over the salad and toss to combine.
4. Serve immediately or chill in the refrigerator for 20 minutes before serving.

TIPS:
- Use fresh lime juice for the best flavor.
- Add a pinch of red pepper flakes for a spicy kick.

N.V.: Calories: 220, Fat: 12g, Carbs: 25g, Protein: 6g, Sugar: 4g, Sodium: 240 mg, Potassium: 600 mg, Cholesterol: 0 mg

MEDITERRANEAN LENTIL SALAD

PREPARATION TIME: 10 min
COOKING TIME: 20 min
MODE OF COOKING: Stovetop
SERVINGS: 4
INGREDIENTS:

- 1 cup green lentils, rinsed
- 3 cups water
- 1 cup cherry tomatoes, halved
- 1/2 cup cucumber, diced
- 1/4 cup red onion, diced
- 1/4 cup Kalamata olives, sliced
- 1/4 cup feta cheese, crumbled
- 2 Tbsp olive oil
- 2 Tbsp red wine vinegar
- 1 tsp dried oregano
- Salt and pepper to taste

DIRECTIONS:

1. In a medium saucepan, bring lentils and water to a boil.
2. Reduce heat to low and simmer for 20 minutes or until lentils are tender but not mushy.
3. Drain and rinse lentils under cold water.
4. In a large bowl, combine cooked lentils, cherry tomatoes, cucumber, red onion, Kalamata olives, and feta cheese.
5. In a small bowl, whisk together olive oil, red wine vinegar, oregano, salt, and pepper.
6. Pour the dressing over the salad and toss to combine.
7. Serve immediately or refrigerate until ready to serve.

TIPS:

- Use French green lentils (Puy lentils) for better texture.
- Add a handful of fresh parsley for added freshness.

N.V.: Calories: 250, Fat: 12g, Carbs: 28g, Protein: 10g, Sugar: 4g, Sodium: 400 mg, Potassium: 600 mg, Cholesterol: 15 mg

GRILLED CHICKEN AND ARUGULA SALAD

PREPARATION TIME: 10 min
COOKING TIME: 10 min
MODE OF COOKING: Grilling
SERVINGS: 4
INGREDIENTS:

- 2 chicken breasts
- 4 cups arugula
- 1/2 cup cherry tomatoes, halved
- 1/4 cup red onion, thinly sliced
- 1/4 cup Parmesan cheese, shaved
- 2 Tbsp olive oil
- 2 Tbsp balsamic vinegar
- 1 tsp Dijon mustard
- Salt and pepper to taste

DIRECTIONS:

1. Preheat grill to medium-high heat.
2. Season chicken breasts with salt and pepper.
3. Grill chicken for 5-7 minutes on each side until fully cooked.
4. Remove chicken from grill and let rest for 5 minutes, then slice thinly.
5. In a large bowl, combine arugula, cherry tomatoes, red onion, and Parmesan cheese.
6. In a small bowl, whisk together olive oil, balsamic vinegar, Dijon mustard, salt, and pepper.
7. Pour the dressing over the salad and toss to combine.
8. Top with sliced grilled chicken.
9. Serve immediately.

TIPS:

- Marinate the chicken in olive oil, lemon juice, and garlic for extra flavor.
- Add roasted red peppers for additional color and taste.

N.V.: Calories: 350, Fat: 18g, Carbs: 10g, Protein: 36g, Sugar: 4g, Sodium: 400 mg, Potassium: 700 mg, Cholesterol: 90 mg

BEET AND GOAT CHEESE SALAD

PREPARATION TIME: 15 min
COOKING TIME: 30 min
MODE OF COOKING: Roasting
SERVINGS: 4
INGREDIENTS:

- 3 medium beets, scrubbed and trimmed
- 4 cups mixed greens (arugula, spinach, etc.)
- 1/4 cup goat cheese, crumbled
- 1/4 cup walnuts, toasted
- 2 Tbsp olive oil
- 2 Tbsp balsamic vinegar
- 1 tsp honey
- Salt and pepper to taste

DIRECTIONS:

1. Preheat oven to 400°F (204°C).
2. Wrap beets in aluminum foil and roast for 30-40 minutes until tender.
3. Let beets cool, then peel and cut into wedges.
4. In a large bowl, combine mixed greens, roasted beets, goat cheese, and toasted walnuts.
5. In a small bowl, whisk together olive oil, balsamic vinegar, honey, salt, and pepper.
6. Pour the dressing over the salad and toss to combine.
7. Serve immediately.

TIPS:

- Wear gloves to avoid staining your hands when peeling beets.
- Add orange segments for a refreshing citrus flavor.

N.V.: Calories: 280, Fat: 18g, Carbs: 23g, Protein: 8g, Sugar: 15g, Sodium: 240 mg, Potassium: 700 mg, Cholesterol: 10 mg

4.2 DIGESTION-FRIENDLY SANDWICHES AND WRAPS: EASY OPTIONS FOR A QUICK LUNCH.

TURKEY AND AVOCADO WRAP

PREPARATION TIME: 10 min
COOKING TIME: N/A
MODE OF COOKING: N/A
SERVINGS: 2
INGREDIENTS:

- 2 whole wheat tortillas
- 6 slices of turkey breast
- 1 avocado, sliced
- 1 cup baby spinach
- 1/2 cup cucumber, sliced
- 1/4 cup hummus
- 1 Tbsp lemon juice
- Salt and pepper to taste

DIRECTIONS:

1. Lay the whole wheat tortillas on a flat surface.
2. Spread hummus evenly over each tortilla.
3. Layer turkey slices, avocado, baby spinach, and cucumber on each tortilla.
4. Drizzle with lemon juice and season with salt and pepper.
5. Roll up the tortillas tightly and slice in half.
6. Serve immediately.

TIPS:

- Use a toothpick to secure the wrap if needed.
- Add a sprinkle of red pepper flakes for extra flavor.

N.V.: Calories: 320, Fat: 15g, Carbs: 34g, Protein: 18g, Sugar: 3g, Sodium: 580 mg, Potassium: 700 mg, Cholesterol: 30 mg

MEDITERRANEAN VEGGIE SANDWICH

PREPARATION TIME: 10 min
COOKING TIME: N/A
MODE OF COOKING: N/A
SERVINGS: 2
INGREDIENTS:

- 4 slices whole grain bread
- 1/2 cup hummus
- 1/2 cup roasted red peppers, sliced
- 1/2 cucumber, sliced
- 1/4 cup Kalamata olives, sliced
- 1/4 cup red onion, thinly sliced
- 1/4 cup feta cheese, crumbled
- 1 cup mixed greens
- 1 Tbsp olive oil
- 1 Tbsp balsamic vinegar
- Salt and pepper to taste

DIRECTIONS:

1. Spread hummus evenly on each slice of bread.
2. Layer roasted red peppers, cucumber, Kalamata olives, red onion, and feta cheese on two slices of bread.
3. Top with mixed greens.
4. Drizzle with olive oil and balsamic vinegar, then season with salt and pepper.
5. Place the remaining bread slices on top to form sandwiches.
6. Serve immediately.

TIPS:

- Grill the sandwich for a warm, melty version.
- Add fresh basil leaves for extra flavor.

N.V.: Calories: 350, Fat: 16g, Carbs: 40g, Protein: 10g, Sugar: 6g, Sodium: 750 mg, Potassium: 400 mg, Cholesterol: 15 mg

CHICKEN AND SPINACH WRAP

PREPARATION TIME: 10 min
COOKING TIME: N/A
MODE OF COOKING: N/A
SERVINGS: 2
INGREDIENTS:

- 2 whole wheat tortillas
- 1 cup cooked chicken breast, shredded
- 1 cup baby spinach
- 1/2 cup cherry tomatoes, halved
- 1/4 cup shredded carrots
- 1/4 cup Greek yogurt
- 1 Tbsp lemon juice
- 1 tsp Dijon mustard
- Salt and pepper to taste

DIRECTIONS:

1. Lay the whole wheat tortillas on a flat surface.
2. In a small bowl, mix Greek yogurt, lemon juice, Dijon mustard, salt, and pepper.
3. Spread the yogurt mixture evenly over each tortilla.
4. Layer shredded chicken, baby spinach, cherry tomatoes, and shredded carrots on each tortilla.
5. Roll up the tortillas tightly and slice in half.
6. Serve immediately.

TIPS:

- Use leftover grilled chicken for extra flavor.
- Add a pinch of paprika for a bit of spice.

N.V.: Calories: 300, Fat: 8g, Carbs: 32g, Protein: 30g, Sugar: 4g, Sodium: 400 mg, Potassium: 700 mg, Cholesterol: 70 mg

TUNA AND AVOCADO SANDWICH

PREPARATION TIME: 10 min
COOKING TIME: N/A
MODE OF COOKING: N/A
SERVINGS: 2
INGREDIENTS:

- 4 slices whole grain bread
- 1 can tuna, drained
- 1 avocado, mashed
- 1/4 cup Greek yogurt
- 1 Tbsp lemon juice
- 1/4 cup celery, diced
- 1/4 cup red onion, diced
- Salt and pepper to taste

DIRECTIONS:

1. In a medium bowl, mix tuna, mashed avocado, Greek yogurt, lemon juice, celery, and red onion.
2. Season with salt and pepper.
3. Spread the tuna mixture evenly on two slices of bread.
4. Top with remaining bread slices to form sandwiches.
5. Serve immediately.

TIPS:

- Add a handful of arugula for extra greens.
- Use a multigrain or sprouted bread for added nutrients.

N.V.: Calories: 330, Fat: 15g, Carbs: 32g, Protein: 22g, Sugar: 3g, Sodium: 500 mg, Potassium: 600 mg, Cholesterol: 30 mg

HUMMUS AND VEGGIE WRAP

PREPARATION TIME: 10 min
COOKING TIME: N/A
MODE OF COOKING: N/A
SERVINGS: 2
INGREDIENTS:
- 2 whole wheat tortillas
- 1/2 cup hummus
- 1/2 cucumber, sliced
- 1/2 red bell pepper, sliced
- 1/4 cup shredded carrots
- 1/4 cup red cabbage, shredded
- 1/4 cup feta cheese, crumbled
- 1 Tbsp lemon juice
- Salt and pepper to taste

DIRECTIONS:
1. Lay the whole wheat tortillas on a flat surface.
2. Spread hummus evenly over each tortilla.
3. Layer cucumber, red bell pepper, shredded carrots, and red cabbage on each tortilla.
4. Sprinkle with feta cheese and drizzle with lemon juice.
5. Season with salt and pepper.
6. Roll up the tortillas tightly and slice in half.
7. Serve immediately.

TIPS:
- Add a few fresh mint leaves for a refreshing flavor.
- Use roasted red peppers for a smoky taste.

N.V.: Calories: 300, Fat: 12g, Carbs: 38g, Protein: 10g, Sugar: 6g, Sodium: 450 mg, Potassium: 500 mg, Cholesterol: 15 mg

4.3 SOOTHING SOUPS AND BROTHS: WARM, COMFORTING RECIPES FOR GUT HEALTH.

GINGER CARROT SOUP

PREPARATION TIME: 15 min
COOKING TIME: 30 min
MODE OF COOKING: Stovetop
SERVINGS: 4
INGREDIENTS:
- 1 lb. carrots, peeled and chopped
- 1 onion, chopped
- 2 cloves garlic, minced
- 1 Tbsp fresh ginger, grated
- 4 cups vegetable broth
- 1 cup coconut milk
- 2 Tbsp olive oil
- Salt and pepper to taste
- Fresh parsley for garnish

DIRECTIONS:
1. In a large pot, heat olive oil over medium heat.
2. Add chopped onions and sauté until translucent, about 5 minutes.
3. Add garlic and ginger, and sauté for another 2 minutes.
4. Add the chopped carrots and vegetable broth. Bring to a boil.
5. Reduce heat and simmer until carrots are tender, about 20 minutes.
6. Using an immersion blender, puree the soup until smooth. Alternatively, transfer the soup in batches to a blender and puree.
7. Stir in coconut milk and season with salt and pepper.
8. Heat through and serve garnished with fresh parsley.

TIPS:
- Add a pinch of turmeric for additional anti-inflammatory benefits.
- Serve with a slice of whole grain bread for a complete meal.

N.V.: Calories: 210, Fat: 14g, Carbs: 21g, Protein: 3g, Sugar: 10g, Sodium: 600 mg, Potassium: 600 mg, Cholesterol: 0 mg

CHICKEN AND RICE SOUP

PREPARATION TIME: 15 min
COOKING TIME: 45 min
MODE OF COOKING: Stovetop
SERVINGS: 4
INGREDIENTS:
- 1 cup cooked chicken breast, shredded
- 1/2 cup brown rice
- 1 onion, chopped
- 2 carrots, chopped
- 2 celery stalks, chopped
- 3 cloves garlic, minced
- 6 cups chicken broth

- 1 bay leaf
- 2 Tbsp olive oil
- Salt and pepper to taste
- Fresh parsley for garnish

DIRECTIONS:
1. In a large pot, heat olive oil over medium heat.
2. Add onions, carrots, and celery, and sauté until vegetables are tender, about 10 minutes.
3. Add garlic and cook for another minute.
4. Pour in chicken broth and add the bay leaf. Bring to a boil.
5. Add the brown rice and reduce heat to a simmer. Cook until rice is tender, about 30 minutes.
6. Stir in the shredded chicken and cook until heated through, about 5 minutes.
7. Season with salt and pepper.
8. Serve garnished with fresh parsley.

TIPS:
- Use leftover roasted chicken for added flavor.
- Add a squeeze of lemon juice for a fresh taste.

N.V.: Calories: 250, Fat: 10g, Carbs: 20g, Protein: 18g, Sugar: 4g, Sodium: 700 mg, Potassium: 500 mg, Cholesterol: 40 mg

BUTTERNUT SQUASH AND APPLE SOUP

PREPARATION TIME: 15 min
COOKING TIME: 30 min
MODE OF COOKING: Stovetop
SERVINGS: 4
INGREDIENTS:
- 1 large butternut squash, peeled and cubed
- 2 apples, peeled, cored, and chopped
- 1 onion, chopped
- 2 cloves garlic, minced
- 4 cups vegetable broth
- 1 cup apple cider
- 2 Tbsp olive oil
- 1/2 tsp ground cinnamon
- Salt and pepper to taste
- Fresh sage for garnish

DIRECTIONS:
1. In a large pot, heat olive oil over medium heat.

2. Add chopped onions and sauté until translucent, about 5 minutes.
3. Add garlic and cook for another minute.
4. Add the cubed butternut squash and chopped apples. Sauté for 5 minutes.
5. Pour in vegetable broth and apple cider. Bring to a boil.
6. Reduce heat and simmer until squash and apples are tender, about 20 minutes.
7. Using an immersion blender, puree the soup until smooth. Alternatively, transfer the soup in batches to a blender and puree.
8. Stir in ground cinnamon and season with salt and pepper.
9. Heat through and serve garnished with fresh sage.

TIPS:
- Add a pinch of nutmeg for additional warmth.
- Serve with a dollop of Greek yogurt for added creaminess.

N.V.: Calories: 190, Fat: 6g, Carbs: 35g, Protein: 2g, Sugar: 18g, Sodium: 400 mg, Potassium: 700 mg, Cholesterol: 0 mg

MISO SOUP WITH TOFU AND SEAWEED

PREPARATION TIME: 10 min
COOKING TIME: 10 min
MODE OF COOKING: Stovetop
SERVINGS: 4
INGREDIENTS:
- 4 cups water
- 1/4 cup miso paste
- 1 cup tofu, cubed
- 1/4 cup wakame seaweed, soaked and drained
- 2 green onions, sliced
- 1/2 cup mushrooms, sliced

DIRECTIONS:
1. In a medium pot, bring water to a gentle simmer.
2. Add miso paste and stir until completely dissolved.
3. Add tofu, soaked seaweed, green onions, and mushrooms.
4. Simmer for 5 minutes until tofu is heated through and mushrooms are tender.

5. Serve immediately.

TIPS:
- Use white miso for a milder flavor or red miso for a stronger taste.
- Add a few slices of ginger for additional warmth.

N.V.: Calories: 70, Fat: 3g, Carbs: 7g, Protein: 5g, Sugar: 2g, Sodium: 750 mg, Potassium: 300 mg, Cholesterol: 0 mg

---

LENTIL AND SPINACH SOUP

PREPARATION TIME: 15 min
COOKING TIME: 30 min
MODE OF COOKING: Stovetop
SERVINGS: 4
INGREDIENTS:
- 1 cup green lentils, rinsed
- 1 onion, chopped
- 2 carrots, chopped
- 2 celery stalks, chopped
- 3 cloves garlic, minced
- 6 cups vegetable broth
- 2 cups baby spinach
- 2 Tbsp olive oil
- 1 tsp cumin
- Salt and pepper to taste
- Fresh cilantro for garnish

DIRECTIONS:
1. In a large pot, heat olive oil over medium heat.
2. Add onions, carrots, and celery, and sauté until vegetables are tender, about 10 minutes.
3. Add garlic and cumin, and cook for another minute.
4. Pour in vegetable broth and add the lentils. Bring to a boil.
5. Reduce heat and simmer until lentils are tender, about 20 minutes.
6. Stir in baby spinach and cook until wilted, about 2 minutes.
7. Season with salt and pepper.
8. Serve garnished with fresh cilantro.

TIPS:
- Add a squeeze of lemon juice for a bright finish.
- Serve with whole grain bread for a hearty meal.

N.V.: Calories: 220, Fat: 7g, Carbs: 30g, Protein: 10g, Sugar: 6g, Sodium: 500 mg, Potassium: 700 mg, Cholesterol: 0 mg

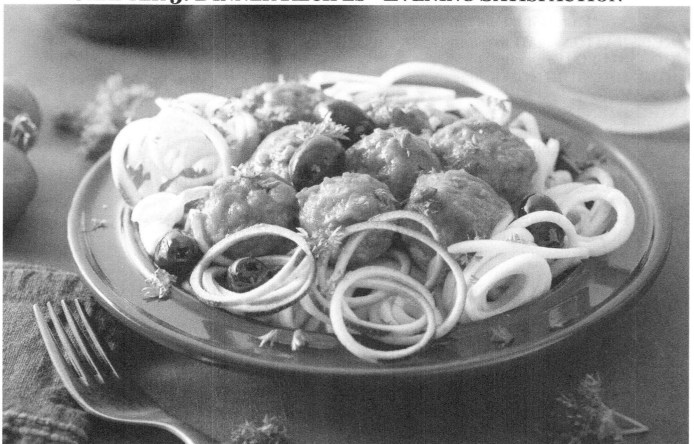

As the sun dips below the horizon and the hustle of the day begins to fade, we find ourselves longing for a moment of tranquility and satisfaction. Dinner is that cherished time when we can unwind, reflect on the day's events, and share a meal with loved ones. It's a ritual that marks the end of the day, offering comfort and nourishment that goes beyond the mere act of eating.

Imagine walking into a kitchen filled with the tantalizing aroma of a slow-cooked stew, the warmth of the stove creating a cozy haven from the outside world. Dinner is not just a meal; it's an experience that brings people together, fostering connection and conversation. Whether it's a simple, quick-to-prepare dish after a long day at work or a more elaborate meal for a special occasion, dinner has the power to transform our evenings into something truly special.

In this chapter, we explore a range of dinner recipes designed to satisfy both the palate and the soul. These recipes cater to a variety of tastes and dietary needs, ensuring that there is something for everyone. From lean proteins and light entrees that offer a healthful end to the day, to comforting one-pot meals that minimize effort while maximizing flavor, you'll find inspiration for every evening.

You'll discover the joy of creating dishes that are not only delicious but also nourishing, helping you to wind down and recharge for the next day. Imagine a plate of perfectly roasted vegetables, their natural sweetness enhanced by a drizzle of balsamic glaze, or a tender piece of grilled fish, seasoned to perfection and served with a refreshing side salad. These recipes are crafted to provide a balance of flavors and textures, making each dinner a memorable occasion.

As you journey through these pages, you'll find tips and tricks to make dinner preparation easier and more enjoyable. Embrace the evening as a time to slow down, savor the process of cooking, and indulge in the satisfaction of a well-prepared meal. Let dinner be your daily reward, a moment of evening satisfaction that nourishes both body and spirit.

LEMON HERB GRILLED CHICKEN	BAKED SALMON WITH DILL

LEMON HERB GRILLED CHICKEN

PREPARATION TIME: 10 min
COOKING TIME: 15 min
MODE OF COOKING: Grilling
SERVINGS: 4
INGREDIENTS:

- 4 boneless, skinless chicken breasts
- 2 Tbsp olive oil
- 2 Tbsp lemon juice
- 2 cloves garlic, minced
- 1 tsp dried oregano
- 1 tsp dried thyme
- Salt and pepper to taste
- Fresh parsley for garnish

DIRECTIONS:

1. In a small bowl, mix olive oil, lemon juice, garlic, oregano, thyme, salt, and pepper.
2. Place chicken breasts in a resealable plastic bag or shallow dish and pour the marinade over the chicken. Marinate for at least 30 minutes.
3. Preheat grill to medium-high heat.
4. Grill chicken breasts for 6-7 minutes per side, or until fully cooked and juices run clear.
5. Remove from grill and let rest for 5 minutes before serving.
6. Garnish with fresh parsley.

TIPS:

- Use fresh herbs for a more intense flavor.
- Pair with a side of steamed vegetables or a green salad.

N.V.: Calories: 220, Fat: 8g, Carbs: 1g, Protein: 34g, Sugar: 0g, Sodium: 150 mg, Potassium: 500 mg, Cholesterol: 85 mg

BAKED SALMON WITH DILL

PREPARATION TIME: 10 min
COOKING TIME: 20 min
MODE OF COOKING: Baking
SERVINGS: 4
INGREDIENTS:

- 4 salmon fillets
- 2 Tbsp olive oil
- 1 Tbsp lemon juice
- 2 tsp dried dill
- Salt and pepper to taste
- Lemon wedges for serving

DIRECTIONS:

1. Preheat oven to 375°F (190°C).
2. In a small bowl, mix olive oil, lemon juice, dill, salt, and pepper.
3. Place salmon fillets on a baking sheet lined with parchment paper.
4. Brush the olive oil mixture over the salmon fillets.
5. Bake for 18-20 minutes, or until salmon is cooked through and flakes easily with a fork.
6. Serve with lemon wedges.

TIPS:

- Add a side of quinoa or brown rice for a complete meal.
- Garnish with fresh dill for extra flavor.

N.V.: Calories: 250, Fat: 14g, Carbs: 0g, Protein: 28g, Sugar: 0g, Sodium: 200 mg, Potassium: 600 mg, Cholesterol: 70 mg

QUINOA-STUFFED BELL PEPPERS

PREPARATION TIME: 15 min
COOKING TIME: 30 min
MODE OF COOKING: Baking
SERVINGS: 4
INGREDIENTS:

- 4 large bell peppers, tops cut off and seeds removed
- 1 cup quinoa, rinsed
- 2 cups vegetable broth
- 1 cup black beans, rinsed and drained
- 1 cup corn kernels
- 1 cup cherry tomatoes, halved
- 1/2 cup red onion, diced
- 1 tsp cumin
- 1 tsp paprika
- Salt and pepper to taste
- 1/4 cup cilantro, chopped
- 1/4 cup shredded cheese (optional)

DIRECTIONS:

1. Preheat oven to 375°F (190°C).
2. In a medium saucepan, bring quinoa and vegetable broth to a boil. Reduce heat and simmer for 15 minutes, or until quinoa is tender and liquid is absorbed.
3. In a large bowl, combine cooked quinoa, black beans, corn, cherry tomatoes, red onion, cumin, paprika, salt, and pepper.
4. Stuff each bell pepper with the quinoa mixture and place them in a baking dish.
5. Cover with foil and bake for 25 minutes.
6. If using, remove foil, sprinkle with shredded cheese, and bake for an additional 5 minutes.
7. Garnish with chopped cilantro before serving.

TIPS:

- Serve with a side of mixed greens for added freshness.
- Use different colored bell peppers for a vibrant presentation.

N.V.: Calories: 280, Fat: 8g, Carbs: 42g, Protein: 10g, Sugar: 8g, Sodium: 350 mg, Potassium: 750 mg, Cholesterol: 0 mg

TURKEY MEATBALLS WITH ZUCCHINI NOODLES

PREPARATION TIME: 15 min
COOKING TIME: 20 min
MODE OF COOKING: Stovetop/Baking
SERVINGS: 4
INGREDIENTS:

- 1 lb. ground turkey
- 1/4 cup breadcrumbs
- 1/4 cup grated Parmesan cheese
- 1 egg
- 2 cloves garlic, minced
- 1 tsp dried oregano
- 1 tsp dried basil
- Salt and pepper to taste
- 2 Tbsp olive oil
- 4 large zucchinis, spiralized
- 1 cup marinara sauce

DIRECTIONS:

1. Preheat oven to 400°F (200°C).
2. In a large bowl, combine ground turkey, breadcrumbs, Parmesan cheese, egg, garlic, oregano, basil, salt, and pepper. Mix well.
3. Form the mixture into meatballs, about 1 inch in diameter.
4. Place meatballs on a baking sheet lined with parchment paper and bake for 15-20 minutes, or until cooked through.
5. In a large skillet, heat olive oil over medium heat. Add spiralized zucchini and sauté for 3-4 minutes, until tender.
6. Serve meatballs over zucchini noodles and top with marinara sauce.

TIPS:

- Substitute ground turkey with ground chicken or lean beef if desired.
- Garnish with fresh basil for added flavor.

N.V.: Calories: 320, Fat: 14g, Carbs: 20g, Protein: 28g, Sugar: 6g, Sodium: 450 mg, Potassium: 900 mg, Cholesterol: 85 mg

BAKED COD WITH LEMON AND HERBS

PREPARATION TIME: 10 min
COOKING TIME: 20 min
MODE OF COOKING: Baking
SERVINGS: 4
INGREDIENTS:
- 4 cod fillets
- 2 Tbsp olive oil
- 2 Tbsp lemon juice
- 2 cloves garlic, minced
- 1 tsp dried thyme
- 1 tsp dried parsley
- Salt and pepper to taste
- Lemon slices for serving

DIRECTIONS:
1. Preheat oven to 375°F (190°C).
2. In a small bowl, mix olive oil, lemon juice, garlic, thyme, parsley, salt, and pepper.
3. Place cod fillets on a baking sheet lined with parchment paper.
4. Brush the olive oil mixture over the cod fillets.
5. Bake for 15-20 minutes, or until cod is cooked through and flakes easily with a fork.
6. Serve with lemon slices.

TIPS:
- Serve with a side of steamed asparagus or roasted vegetables.
- Add a sprinkle of red pepper flakes for a hint of spice.

N.V.: Calories: 220, Fat: 10g, Carbs: 2g, Protein: 28g, Sugar: 0g, Sodium: 200 mg, Potassium: 600 mg, Cholesterol: 70 mg

•5.2 COMFORTING ONE-POT MEALS: MINIMAL EFFORT FOR MAXIMUM FLAVOR.

ONE-POT CHICKEN AND RICE

PREPARATION TIME: 10 min
COOKING TIME: 30 min
MODE OF COOKING: Stovetop
SERVINGS: 4
INGREDIENTS:
- 4 boneless, skinless chicken thighs
- 1 cup long-grain rice
- 2 cups chicken broth
- 1 onion, chopped
- 2 cloves garlic, minced
- 1 cup peas
- 1 cup carrots, chopped
- 1 Tbsp olive oil
- 1 tsp paprika
- 1 tsp dried thyme
- Salt and pepper to taste
- Fresh parsley for garnish

DIRECTIONS:
1. In a large pot, heat olive oil over medium heat.
2. Season chicken thighs with salt, pepper, paprika, and thyme.
3. Add chicken to the pot and brown on both sides, about 4-5 minutes per side. Remove chicken and set aside.
4. In the same pot, add chopped onion and garlic. Sauté until translucent, about 3 minutes.
5. Add rice and cook for 2 minutes, stirring constantly.
6. Pour in chicken broth and bring to a boil.
7. Return chicken thighs to the pot, cover, and reduce heat to low. Simmer for 20 minutes.
8. Add peas and carrots, cover, and cook for an additional 5 minutes until vegetables are tender.
9. Serve garnished with fresh parsley.

TIPS:
- Use bone-in chicken thighs for more flavor.
- Substitute with brown rice for added fiber.

N.V.: Calories: 350, Fat: 12g, Carbs: 36g, Protein: 22g, Sugar: 4g, Sodium: 600 mg, Potassium: 600 mg, Cholesterol: 70 mg

ONE-POT PASTA PRIMAVERA

PREPARATION TIME: 10 min
COOKING TIME: 20 min
MODE OF COOKING: Stovetop
SERVINGS: 4
INGREDIENTS:

- 12 oz whole wheat pasta
- 1 zucchini, sliced
- 1 bell pepper, sliced
- 1 cup cherry tomatoes, halved
- 1 cup broccoli florets
- 3 cloves garlic, minced
- 4 cups vegetable broth
- 1/4 cup Parmesan cheese, grated
- 2 Tbsp olive oil
- Salt and pepper to taste
- Fresh basil for garnish

DIRECTIONS:

1. In a large pot, heat olive oil over medium heat.
2. Add minced garlic and sauté for 1 minute.
3. Add sliced zucchini, bell pepper, cherry tomatoes, and broccoli. Sauté for 3-4 minutes until vegetables begin to soften.
4. Add whole wheat pasta and vegetable broth. Bring to a boil.
5. Reduce heat and simmer, stirring occasionally, until pasta is cooked and liquid is absorbed, about 12-15 minutes.
6. Stir in grated Parmesan cheese.
7. Season with salt and pepper to taste.
8. Serve garnished with fresh basil.

TIPS:

- Add a pinch of red pepper flakes for a bit of heat.
- Substitute Parmesan with nutritional yeast for a dairy-free option.

N.V.: Calories: 320, Fat: 10g, Carbs: 50g, Protein: 12g, Sugar: 6g, Sodium: 400 mg, Potassium: 700 mg, Cholesterol: 10 mg

ONE-POT BEEF AND VEGETABLE STEW

PREPARATION TIME: 15 min
COOKING TIME: 1 hr.
MODE OF COOKING: Stovetop
SERVINGS: 4
INGREDIENTS:

- 1 lb. beef stew meat, cubed
- 2 potatoes, cubed
- 3 carrots, sliced
- 2 celery stalks, chopped
- 1 onion, chopped
- 3 cloves garlic, minced
- 4 cups beef broth
- 1 Tbsp tomato paste
- 1 tsp dried thyme
- 1 tsp dried rosemary
- 2 Tbsp olive oil
- Salt and pepper to taste
- Fresh parsley for garnish

DIRECTIONS:

1. In a large pot, heat olive oil over medium-high heat.
2. Season beef stew meat with salt and pepper.
3. Brown the beef in batches, then remove and set aside.
4. In the same pot, add chopped onion, garlic, carrots, and celery. Sauté until vegetables are tender, about 5 minutes.
5. Add tomato paste and cook for 1 minute.
6. Return beef to the pot and add potatoes, beef broth, thyme, and rosemary. Bring to a boil.
7. Reduce heat to low, cover, and simmer for 1 hour until beef is tender.
8. Season with salt and pepper to taste.
9. Serve garnished with fresh parsley.

TIPS:

- Use a slow cooker for an even more tender stew.
- Serve with crusty bread for a complete meal.

N.V.: Calories: 380, Fat: 18g, Carbs: 30g, Protein: 25g, Sugar: 6g, Sodium: 600 mg, Potassium: 800 mg, Cholesterol: 70 mg

ONE-POT CHICKEN AND QUINOA

PREPARATION TIME: 10 min
COOKING TIME: 30 min
MODE OF COOKING: Stovetop
SERVINGS: 4
INGREDIENTS:

- 4 boneless, skinless chicken breasts
- 1 cup quinoa, rinsed
- 2 cups chicken broth
- 1 onion, chopped
- 2 cloves garlic, minced
- 1 bell pepper, chopped
- 1 cup spinach, chopped
- 1 tsp paprika
- 1 tsp cumin
- 2 Tbsp olive oil
- Salt and pepper to taste
- Fresh cilantro for garnish

DIRECTIONS:

1. In a large pot, heat olive oil over medium heat.
2. Season chicken breasts with salt, pepper, paprika, and cumin.
3. Add chicken to the pot and brown on both sides, about 4-5 minutes per side. Remove chicken and set aside.
4. In the same pot, add chopped onion, garlic, and bell pepper. Sauté until tender, about 5 minutes.
5. Add quinoa and chicken broth. Bring to a boil.
6. Return chicken breasts to the pot, cover, and reduce heat to low. Simmer for 20 minutes.
7. Stir in chopped spinach and cook until wilted, about 2 minutes.
8. Serve garnished with fresh cilantro.

TIPS:

- Use chicken thighs for a juicier option.
- Add a squeeze of lime juice for a fresh finish.

N.V.: Calories: 320, Fat: 10g, Carbs: 28g, Protein: 34g, Sugar: 4g, Sodium: 500 mg, Potassium: 700 mg, Cholesterol: 85 mg

ONE-POT MEDITERRANEAN SHRIMP AND ORZO

PREPARATION TIME: 10 min
COOKING TIME: 20 min
MODE OF COOKING: Stovetop
SERVINGS: 4
INGREDIENTS:

- 1 lb. shrimp, peeled and deveined
- 1 cup orzo
- 2 cups vegetable broth
- 1 cup cherry tomatoes, halved
- 1/2 cup Kalamata olives, sliced
- 1/4 cup red onion, chopped
- 3 cloves garlic, minced
- 2 Tbsp olive oil
- 1 tsp dried oregano
- Salt and pepper to taste
- Fresh parsley for garnish
- Lemon wedges for serving

DIRECTIONS:

1. In a large pot, heat olive oil over medium heat.
2. Add chopped red onion and garlic. Sauté until translucent, about 3 minutes.
3. Add orzo and cook for 2 minutes, stirring constantly.
4. Pour in vegetable broth and bring to a boil.
5. Reduce heat and simmer for 10 minutes.
6. Add shrimp, cherry tomatoes, and Kalamata olives. Cook until shrimp is pink and opaque, about 5 minutes.
7. Season with oregano, salt, and pepper.
8. Serve garnished with fresh parsley and lemon wedges.

TIPS:

- Use whole wheat orzo for added fiber.
- Add spinach or arugula for extra greens.

N.V.: Calories: 340, Fat: 12g, Carbs: 34g, Protein: 24g, Sugar: 4g, Sodium: 600 mg, Potassium: 500 mg, Cholesterol: 150 mg

STUFFED BELL PEPPERS WITH QUINOA AND BLACK BEANS

PREPARATION TIME: 15 min
COOKING TIME: 30 min
MODE OF COOKING: Baking
SERVINGS: 4
INGREDIENTS:

- 4 large bell peppers, tops cut off and seeds removed
- 1 cup quinoa, rinsed
- 2 cups vegetable broth
- 1 cup black beans, rinsed and drained
- 1 cup corn kernels
- 1 cup cherry tomatoes, halved
- 1/2 cup red onion, diced
- 1 tsp cumin
- 1 tsp paprika
- Salt and pepper to taste
- 1/4 cup cilantro, chopped
- 1/4 cup vegan cheese (optional)

DIRECTIONS:

1. Preheat oven to 375°F (190°C).
2. In a medium saucepan, bring quinoa and vegetable broth to a boil. Reduce heat and simmer for 15 minutes, or until quinoa is tender and liquid is absorbed.
3. In a large bowl, combine cooked quinoa, black beans, corn, cherry tomatoes, red onion, cumin, paprika, salt, and pepper.
4. Stuff each bell pepper with the quinoa mixture and place them in a baking dish.
5. Cover with foil and bake for 25 minutes.
6. If using, remove foil, sprinkle with vegan cheese, and bake for an additional 5 minutes.
7. Garnish with chopped cilantro before serving.

TIPS:

- Use different colored bell peppers for a vibrant presentation.
- Serve with a side salad for a complete meal.

N.V.: Calories: 290, Fat: 6g, Carbs: 50g, Protein: 10g, Sugar: 8g, Sodium: 350 mg, Potassium: 750 mg, Cholesterol: 0 mg

CHICKPEA AND SPINACH CURRY

PREPARATION TIME: 10 min
COOKING TIME: 20 min
MODE OF COOKING: Stovetop
SERVINGS: 4
INGREDIENTS:

- 1 can chickpeas, rinsed and drained
- 4 cups baby spinach
- 1 onion, chopped
- 2 cloves garlic, minced
- 1 can coconut milk
- 1 can diced tomatoes
- 2 Tbsp curry powder
- 1 tsp ground cumin
- 1 tsp ground coriander
- 1 Tbsp olive oil
- Salt and pepper to taste
- Fresh cilantro for garnish

DIRECTIONS:

1. In a large pot, heat olive oil over medium heat.
2. Add chopped onion and sauté until translucent, about 5 minutes.
3. Add garlic and cook for another minute.
4. Stir in curry powder, cumin, and coriander, and cook for 1 minute until fragrant.
5. Add chickpeas, coconut milk, and diced tomatoes. Bring to a boil.
6. Reduce heat and simmer for 10 minutes.
7. Stir in baby spinach and cook until wilted, about 2 minutes.
8. Season with salt and pepper.
9. Serve garnished with fresh cilantro.

TIPS:

- Serve over brown rice or quinoa.
- Add a squeeze of lime juice for a fresh flavor.

N.V.: Calories: 300, Fat: 16g, Carbs: 34g, Protein: 10g, Sugar: 6g, Sodium: 400 mg, Potassium: 700 mg, Cholesterol: 0 mg

EGGPLANT AND TOMATO STEW

PREPARATION TIME: 10 min
COOKING TIME: 30 min
MODE OF COOKING: Stovetop
SERVINGS: 4
INGREDIENTS:
- 2 large eggplants, cubed
- 1 onion, chopped
- 3 cloves garlic, minced
- 1 can diced tomatoes
- 1 cup vegetable broth
- 1 Tbsp tomato paste
- 1 tsp dried oregano
- 1 tsp dried basil
- 2 Tbsp olive oil
- Salt and pepper to taste
- Fresh basil for garnish

DIRECTIONS:
1. In a large pot, heat olive oil over medium heat.
2. Add chopped onion and sauté until translucent, about 5 minutes.
3. Add garlic and cook for another minute.
4. Stir in tomato paste and cook for 1 minute.
5. Add eggplant, diced tomatoes, vegetable broth, oregano, and basil. Bring to a boil.
6. Reduce heat and simmer until eggplant is tender, about 20 minutes.
7. Season with salt and pepper.
8. Serve garnished with fresh basil.

TIPS:
- Serve with crusty bread or over couscous.
- Add a pinch of red pepper flakes for a bit of heat.

N.V.: Calories: 180, Fat: 10g, Carbs: 24g, Protein: 4g, Sugar: 10g, Sodium: 350 mg, Potassium: 600 mg, Cholesterol: 0 mg

SWEET POTATO AND KALE HASH

PREPARATION TIME: 10 min
COOKING TIME: 20 min
MODE OF COOKING: Stovetop
SERVINGS: 4
INGREDIENTS:
- 2 large sweet potatoes, peeled and cubed
- 4 cups kale, chopped
- 1 red bell pepper, chopped
- 1 onion, chopped
- 2 cloves garlic, minced
- 2 Tbsp olive oil
- 1 tsp smoked paprika
- Salt and pepper to taste
- Fresh parsley for garnish

DIRECTIONS:
1. In a large skillet, heat olive oil over medium heat.
2. Add chopped onion and sauté until translucent, about 5 minutes.
3. Add garlic and cook for another minute.
4. Stir in sweet potatoes, red bell pepper, and smoked paprika. Cook, stirring occasionally, until sweet potatoes are tender, about 15 minutes.
5. Add chopped kale and cook until wilted, about 3 minutes.
6. Season with salt and pepper.
7. Serve garnished with fresh parsley.

TIPS:
- Add a poached egg on top for extra protein.
- Serve with a side of avocado slices.

N.V.: Calories: 250, Fat: 10g, Carbs: 38g, Protein: 4g, Sugar: 8g, Sodium: 300 mg, Potassium: 800 mg, Cholesterol: 0 mg

LENTIL AND VEGETABLE SHEPHERD'S PIE

PREPARATION TIME: 15 min
COOKING TIME: 30 min
MODE OF COOKING: Baking
SERVINGS: 4
INGREDIENTS:

- 1 cup green lentils, rinsed
- 3 cups vegetable broth
- 2 carrots, chopped
- 1 cup peas
- 1 cup corn
- 1 onion, chopped
- 2 cloves garlic, minced
- 2 Tbsp tomato paste
- 1 tsp thyme
- 2 Tbsp olive oil
- 4 cups mashed potatoes
- Salt and pepper to taste

DIRECTIONS:

1. Preheat oven to 375°F (190°C).
2. In a large pot, heat olive oil over medium heat.
3. Add chopped onion and garlic, and sauté until translucent, about 5 minutes.
4. Stir in tomato paste and cook for 1 minute.
5. Add lentils, vegetable broth, carrots, peas, corn, and thyme. Bring to a boil.
6. Reduce heat and simmer until lentils are tender and broth is absorbed, about 20 minutes.
7. Transfer lentil mixture to a baking dish and spread mashed potatoes evenly over the top.
8. Bake for 20 minutes until the top is golden brown.
9. Season with salt and pepper.

TIPS:

- Use sweet potatoes for the mash for a different flavor.
- Add a sprinkle of nutritional yeast on top for a cheesy flavor.

N.V.: Calories: 350, Fat: 12g, Carbs: 50g, Protein: 12g, Sugar: 6g, Sodium: 450 mg, Potassium: 900 mg, Cholesterol: 0 mg

CHAPTER 6: SNACKS AND SMALL BITES

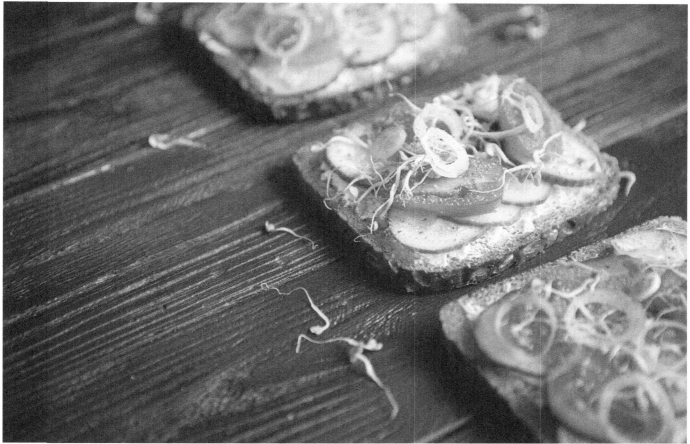

In the rhythm of our daily lives, it's often the small moments that bring the most joy. Amid the hustle and bustle, snacks and small bites serve as delightful interludes, offering a burst of energy, a touch of comfort, or simply a moment to savor something delicious. These little indulgences bridge the gaps between our main meals, ensuring that we remain nourished and satisfied throughout the day.

Picture a mid-morning break with a handful of freshly roasted nuts, their warmth and crunch providing a satisfying contrast to the day's activities. Or imagine a late-afternoon pause with a refreshing smoothie, its vibrant colors and flavors revitalizing your senses. Snacks are not just fillers; they are essential components of our daily nutrition, helping to maintain our energy levels and keep hunger at bay.

In this chapter, we celebrate the art of snacking with a collection of recipes that are as nourishing as they are enjoyable. From quick, healthy snacks that can be whipped up in minutes, to more elaborate small bites perfect for entertaining, these recipes cater to a variety of tastes and dietary needs. Each one is crafted to offer the perfect balance of flavor and nutrition, ensuring that every bite is a pleasure.

You'll discover options that range from crunchy and savory to sweet and satisfying. Think of a plate of crispy kale chips, lightly seasoned and baked to perfection, or a bowl of creamy hummus, paired with colorful vegetable sticks. There's joy in these simple preparations, transforming everyday ingredients into something special.

For those moments when you need a bit of indulgence, you'll find recipes for treats that are still mindful of your health. Imagine biting into a piece of dark chocolate bark, studded with nuts and dried fruits, each piece a little moment of bliss. Or perhaps a batch of homemade granola bars, packed with wholesome ingredients and just the right amount of sweetness.

As you explore these recipes, you'll see that snacking can be both nutritious and delightful. It's about finding that perfect bite that not only satisfies your hunger but also brings a smile to your face. Let these snacks and small bites be your companions throughout the day, adding a touch of joy and nourishment to every moment.

•6.1 QUICK HEALTHY SNACKS: EASY RECIPES FOR BETWEEN-MEAL HUNGER.

APPLE AND ALMOND BUTTER BITES

PREPARATION TIME: 5 min
COOKING TIME: N/A
MODE OF COOKING: N/A
SERVINGS: 2
INGREDIENTS:
- 1 large apple, sliced
- 2 Tbsp almond butter
- 1 Tbsp chia seeds
- 1 Tbsp honey (optional)
- 1/4 tsp cinnamon

DIRECTIONS:
1. Arrange apple slices on a plate.
2. Spread almond butter evenly over each apple slice.
3. Sprinkle with chia seeds and a dash of cinnamon.
4. Drizzle with honey if desired.
5. Serve immediately.

TIPS:
- Use different types of apples for a variety of flavors.
- Substitute almond butter with peanut or cashew butter.

N.V.: Calories: 220, Fat: 12g, Carbs: 26g, Protein: 4g, Sugar: 15g, Sodium: 0 mg, Potassium: 270 mg, Cholesterol: 0 mg

GREEK YOGURT AND BERRY PARFAIT

PREPARATION TIME: 5 min
COOKING TIME: N/A
MODE OF COOKING: N/A
SERVINGS: 2
INGREDIENTS:
- 1 cup Greek yogurt
- 1 cup mixed berries (strawberries, blueberries, raspberries)
- 1/4 cup granola
- 1 Tbsp honey
- 1 tsp vanilla extract

DIRECTIONS:
1. In a bowl, mix Greek yogurt and vanilla extract.
2. Layer yogurt mixture, berries, and granola in serving glasses.
3. Drizzle with honey.
4. Serve immediately.

TIPS:
- Use frozen berries if fresh ones are not available.
- Add a sprinkle of nuts or seeds for extra crunch.

N.V.: Calories: 250, Fat: 8g, Carbs: 32g, Protein: 14g, Sugar: 20g, Sodium: 80 mg, Potassium: 400 mg, Cholesterol: 10 mg

AVOCADO TOAST WITH CHERRY TOMATOES

PREPARATION TIME: 5 min
COOKING TIME: 5 min
MODE OF COOKING: Toasting
SERVINGS: 2
INGREDIENTS:
- 2 slices whole grain bread
- 1 ripe avocado, mashed
- 1/2 cup cherry tomatoes, halved
- 1 Tbsp olive oil
- Salt and pepper to taste
- 1/4 tsp red pepper flakes (optional)

DIRECTIONS:
1. Toast the bread slices until golden brown.
2. Spread mashed avocado evenly over the toast.
3. Top with cherry tomatoes.
4. Drizzle with olive oil and season with salt, pepper, and red pepper flakes if desired.
5. Serve immediately.

TIPS:
- Add a poached egg on top for extra protein.
- Use multigrain bread for added texture and flavor.

N.V.: Calories: 300, Fat: 22g, Carbs: 26g, Protein: 6g, Sugar: 2g, Sodium: 200 mg, Potassium: 600 mg, Cholesterol: 0 mg

HUMMUS AND VEGGIE STICKS

PREPARATION TIME: 10 min
COOKING TIME: N/A
MODE OF COOKING: N/A
SERVINGS: 2
INGREDIENTS:
- 1 cup hummus
- 1 carrot, cut into sticks
- 1 cucumber, cut into sticks
- 1 bell pepper, cut into sticks
- 1 celery stalk, cut into sticks

DIRECTIONS:
1. Arrange the veggie sticks on a plate.
2. Serve with hummus on the side.
3. Enjoy as a dip and snack.

TIPS:
- Use a variety of colored bell peppers for a vibrant presentation.
- Add a sprinkle of paprika or cumin to the hummus for extra flavor.

N.V.: Calories: 180, Fat: 10g, Carbs: 18g, Protein: 6g, Sugar: 5g, Sodium: 300 mg, Potassium: 450 mg, Cholesterol: 0 mg

BANANA AND ALMOND BUTTER ROLL-UPS

PREPARATION TIME: 5 min
COOKING TIME: N/A
MODE OF COOKING: N/A
SERVINGS: 2
INGREDIENTS:
- 2 whole wheat tortillas
- 2 bananas, peeled
- 2 Tbsp almond butter
- 1 Tbsp honey
- 1/2 tsp cinnamon

DIRECTIONS:
1. Lay tortillas flat and spread almond butter evenly over each.
2. Place a banana on each tortilla and drizzle with honey.
3. Sprinkle with cinnamon.
4. Roll up the tortillas tightly and slice into bite-sized pieces.
5. Serve immediately.

TIPS:
- Use a different nut butter for variety.
- Add a sprinkle of chia seeds for extra nutrition.

N.V.: Calories: 250, Fat: 9g, Carbs: 42g, Protein: 6g, Sugar: 16g, Sodium: 150 mg, Potassium: 500 mg, Cholesterol: 0 mg

•6.2 FINGER FOODS FOR DIGESTIVE HEALTH: ENJOYABLE AND GENTLE ON THE STOMACH.

BAKED ZUCCHINI CHIPS

PREPARATION TIME: 10 min
COOKING TIME: 20 min
MODE OF COOKING: Baking
SERVINGS: 4
INGREDIENTS:
- 2 large zucchinis, thinly sliced
- 2 Tbsp olive oil
- 1/2 tsp salt
- 1/4 tsp black pepper
- 1/4 tsp garlic powder
- 1/4 tsp paprika

DIRECTIONS:
1. Preheat oven to 375°F (190°C).
2. In a large bowl, toss zucchini slices with olive oil, salt, pepper, garlic powder, and paprika.
3. Arrange zucchini slices in a single layer on a baking sheet lined with parchment paper.
4. Bake for 15-20 minutes or until crispy and golden brown, turning once halfway through.
5. Allow to cool slightly before serving.

TIPS:
- Use a mandolin slicer for even, thin slices.
- Serve with a yogurt-based dip for extra flavor.

N.V.: Calories: 70, Fat: 5g, Carbs: 6g, Protein: 1g, Sugar: 2g, Sodium: 150 mg, Potassium: 250 mg, Cholesterol: 0 mg

CUCUMBER AND HUMMUS BITES

PREPARATION TIME: 10 min
COOKING TIME: N/A
MODE OF COOKING: N/A
SERVINGS: 4
INGREDIENTS:

- 2 large cucumbers, sliced into rounds
- 1 cup hummus
- 1/4 cup cherry tomatoes, quartered
- 1/4 cup Kalamata olives, sliced
- Fresh dill for garnish

DIRECTIONS:

1. Arrange cucumber rounds on a serving platter.
2. Top each cucumber round with a spoonful of hummus.
3. Garnish with cherry tomatoes, olives, and a sprig of fresh dill.
4. Serve immediately.

TIPS:

- Use different types of hummus for variety.
- Add a sprinkle of feta cheese for extra flavor.

N.V.: Calories: 80, Fat: 4g, Carbs: 8g, Protein: 3g, Sugar: 2g, Sodium: 200 mg, Potassium: 250 mg, Cholesterol: 0 mg

SWEET POTATO TOASTS WITH AVOCADO

PREPARATION TIME: 10 min
COOKING TIME: 15 min
MODE OF COOKING: Baking
SERVINGS: 4
INGREDIENTS:

- 2 large sweet potatoes, sliced lengthwise into 1/4-inch slices
- 2 avocados, mashed
- 1 Tbsp lemon juice
- Salt and pepper to taste
- 1/4 tsp red pepper flakes (optional)
- Olive oil spray

DIRECTIONS:

1. Preheat oven to 375°F (190°C).
2. Arrange sweet potato slices on a baking sheet and lightly spray with olive oil.
3. Bake for 15 minutes or until tender and slightly crispy.
4. In a bowl, mix mashed avocados with lemon juice, salt, and pepper.
5. Spread avocado mixture on sweet potato slices.
6. Sprinkle with red pepper flakes if desired.
7. Serve immediately.

TIPS:

- Top with cherry tomatoes or radish slices for added texture.
- Use a toaster instead of an oven for quicker preparation.

N.V.: Calories: 150, Fat: 9g, Carbs: 18g, Protein: 2g, Sugar: 4g, Sodium: 150 mg, Potassium: 600 mg, Cholesterol: 0 mg

BAKED CARROT FRIES

PREPARATION TIME: 10 min
COOKING TIME: 25 min
MODE OF COOKING: Baking
SERVINGS: 4
INGREDIENTS:

- 6 large carrots, peeled and cut into sticks
- 2 Tbsp olive oil
- 1/2 tsp salt
- 1/4 tsp black pepper
- 1/4 tsp cumin
- 1/4 tsp paprika

DIRECTIONS:

1. Preheat oven to 375°F (190°C).
2. In a large bowl, toss carrot sticks with olive oil, salt, pepper, cumin, and paprika.
3. Arrange carrot sticks in a single layer on a baking sheet lined with parchment paper.
4. Bake for 25 minutes or until tender and slightly crispy, turning once halfway through.
5. Serve immediately.

TIPS:

- Serve with a yogurt dip for extra flavor.
- Add a sprinkle of Parmesan cheese for a cheesy twist.

N.V.: Calories: 90, Fat: 5g, Carbs: 12g, Protein: 1g, Sugar: 6g, Sodium: 200 mg, Potassium: 300 mg, Cholesterol: 0 mg

MINI CAPRESE SKEWERS

PREPARATION TIME: 10 min
COOKING TIME: N/A
MODE OF COOKING: N/A
SERVINGS: 4
INGREDIENTS:

- 1 cup cherry tomatoes
- 1 cup mini mozzarella balls (bocconcini)
- Fresh basil leaves
- 2 Tbsp balsamic glaze
- Toothpicks or small skewers

DIRECTIONS:

1. Thread one cherry tomato, one mini mozzarella ball, and one basil leaf onto each toothpick or skewer.
2. Arrange on a serving platter.
3. Drizzle with balsamic glaze.
4. Serve immediately.

TIPS:

- Use a mix of red and yellow cherry tomatoes for a colorful presentation.
- Add a sprinkle of sea salt for extra flavor.

N.V.: Calories: 110, Fat: 7g, Carbs: 5g, Protein: 6g, Sugar: 4g, Sodium: 150 mg, Potassium: 200 mg, Cholesterol: 15 mg

•6.3 FIBER-RICH SNACKS: OPTIONS TO KEEP DIGESTION SMOOTH.

CHIA PUDDING WITH FRESH BERRIES

PREPARATION TIME: 5 min
COOKING TIME: N/A (Chill for 2 hours)
MODE OF COOKING: N/A
SERVINGS: 2
INGREDIENTS:

- 1/4 cup chia seeds
- 1 cup almond milk
- 1 Tbsp honey
- 1/2 tsp vanilla extract
- 1 cup mixed berries (strawberries, blueberries, raspberries)

DIRECTIONS:

1. In a bowl, combine chia seeds, almond milk, honey, and vanilla extract. Stir well.
2. Cover and refrigerate for at least 2 hours, or overnight, until thickened.
3. Stir the chia pudding once more and divide between two bowls.
4. Top with mixed berries before serving.

TIPS:

- Add a sprinkle of nuts or seeds for extra crunch.
- Substitute almond milk with coconut milk for a creamier texture.

N.V.: Calories: 180, Fat: 8g, Carbs: 26g, Protein: 4g, Sugar: 12g, Sodium: 70 mg, Potassium: 250 mg, Cholesterol: 0 mg

BAKED APPLE CHIPS

PREPARATION TIME: 10 min
COOKING TIME: 2 hr.
MODE OF COOKING: Baking
SERVINGS: 4
INGREDIENTS:

- 2 large apples, thinly sliced
- 1 tsp cinnamon
- 1 Tbsp honey (optional)

DIRECTIONS:

1. Preheat oven to 200°F (93°C).
2. Arrange apple slices in a single layer on a baking sheet lined with parchment paper.
3. Sprinkle with cinnamon and drizzle with honey if desired.
4. Bake for 2 hours, turning once halfway through, until apples are dry and crispy.
5. Let cool before serving.

TIPS:

- Use a mandolin slicer for even slices.
- Store in an airtight container for up to a week.

N.V.: Calories: 60, Fat: 0g, Carbs: 16g, Protein: 0g, Sugar: 12g, Sodium: 0 mg, Potassium: 150 mg, Cholesterol: 0 mg

EDAMAME WITH SEA SALT

PREPARATION TIME: 5 min
COOKING TIME: 10 min
MODE OF COOKING: Boiling
SERVINGS: 4
INGREDIENTS:

- 2 cups edamame (in pods)
- 1 Tbsp sea salt

DIRECTIONS:

1. Bring a pot of water to a boil.
2. Add edamame and boil for 5-6 minutes until tender.
3. Drain and sprinkle with sea salt.
4. Serve warm or chilled.

TIPS:

- Add a squeeze of lemon juice for a zesty flavor.
- Serve with a sprinkle of sesame seeds for added texture.

N.V.: Calories: 120, Fat: 5g, Carbs: 10g, Protein: 11g, Sugar: 2g, Sodium: 350 mg, Potassium: 280 mg, Cholesterol: 0 mg

ROASTED CHICKPEAS

PREPARATION TIME: 5 min
COOKING TIME: 30 min
MODE OF COOKING: Baking
SERVINGS: 4
INGREDIENTS:

- 1 can chickpeas, rinsed and drained
- 1 Tbsp olive oil
- 1/2 tsp smoked paprika
- 1/2 tsp garlic powder
- 1/2 tsp cumin
- Salt and pepper to taste

DIRECTIONS:

1. Preheat oven to 400°F (204°C).
2. Pat chickpeas dry with a paper towel.
3. In a bowl, toss chickpeas with olive oil, smoked paprika, garlic powder, cumin, salt, and pepper.
4. Spread chickpeas in a single layer on a baking sheet.
5. Bake for 30-35 minutes, stirring halfway through, until crispy.
6. Allow to cool before serving.

TIPS:

- Store in an airtight container for up to 3 days.
- Use different spices for variety.

N.V.: Calories: 140, Fat: 6g, Carbs: 18g, Protein: 5g, Sugar: 1g, Sodium: 220 mg, Potassium: 220 mg, Cholesterol: 0 mg

AVOCADO AND BLACK BEAN DIP WITH VEGGIE STICKS

PREPARATION TIME: 10 min
COOKING TIME: N/A
MODE OF COOKING: N/A
SERVINGS: 4
INGREDIENTS:

- 1 avocado, mashed
- 1 cup black beans, rinsed and mashed
- 1/4 cup red onion, finely chopped
- 1 clove garlic, minced
- 1 Tbsp lime juice
- Salt and pepper to taste
- Carrot sticks, celery sticks, bell pepper strips for serving

DIRECTIONS:

1. In a bowl, combine mashed avocado, black beans, red onion, garlic, and lime juice.
2. Season with salt and pepper.
3. Mix until well combined.
4. Serve with carrot sticks, celery sticks, and bell pepper strips.

TIPS:

- Add a sprinkle of cilantro for extra freshness.
- Serve with whole grain crackers as an alternative.

N.V.: Calories: 180, Fat: 8g, Carbs: 22g, Protein: 5g, Sugar: 2g, Sodium: 150 mg, Potassium: 480 mg, Cholesterol: 0 mg

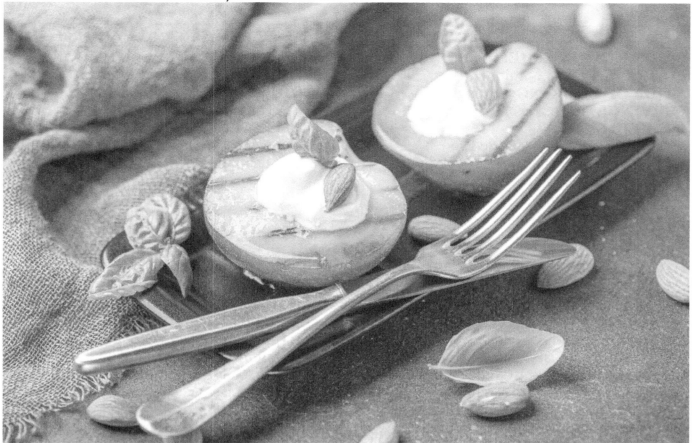

After a day filled with activities and nourishing meals, there comes a moment that many of us anticipate with delight the sweet finale of dessert. Desserts have an almost magical quality, capable of transforming the end of a meal into a memorable experience. They are the punctuation mark to our culinary journey, offering sweetness and satisfaction that lingers.

Imagine sitting down to enjoy a light, fluffy piece of angel food cake, its delicate sweetness enhanced by a dollop of fresh berries. Or picture the soothing warmth of a bowl of baked apples, spiced just right and drizzled with a touch of honey. Desserts, when crafted with care, can be both indulgent and gentle on the palate, satisfying our cravings without overwhelming our senses.

In this chapter, we explore the world of desserts that are both sweet and gentle. These recipes are designed to provide that perfect touch of sweetness while being mindful of ingredients that promote health and well-being. Whether you are seeking to indulge in a rich chocolate mousse or a refreshing fruit sorbet, you will find recipes that cater to a variety of tastes and dietary needs.

We delve into naturally sweetened desserts, where the flavors of fruits and natural sugars take center stage. Think of a luscious peach cobbler that highlights the fruit's natural sweetness or a silky panna cotta infused with vanilla and topped with a fresh berry compote. These desserts are crafted to bring out the best in their ingredients, offering a balance of flavors that is both satisfying and delightful.

Low-fat baking becomes an art in this chapter, where we create treats that allow you to indulge without the guilt. Picture a batch of lemon almond cookies, their crisp edges giving way to a tender center, or a slice of carrot cake, moist and spiced to perfection, topped with a light cream cheese frosting. These recipes show that it's possible to enjoy the richness of dessert while keeping it light.

As you explore these recipes, you'll discover that dessert can be a celebration of flavor, texture, and creativity. It's about finding joy in the sweet moments and sharing them with those you love. Let these desserts be a gentle end to your meals, a sweet note that leaves you satisfied and content.

BANANA OAT COOKIES

PREPARATION TIME: 10 min
COOKING TIME: 15 min
MODE OF COOKING: Baking
SERVINGS: 12 cookies
INGREDIENTS:
- 2 ripe bananas, mashed
- 1 1/2 cups rolled oats
- 1/4 cup almond butter
- 1/4 cup raisins
- 1 tsp vanilla extract
- 1/2 tsp cinnamon
- 1/4 tsp salt

DIRECTIONS:
1. Preheat oven to 350°F (175°C).
2. In a large bowl, mix mashed bananas, almond butter, and vanilla extract until smooth.
3. Add rolled oats, raisins, cinnamon, and salt. Mix until well combined.
4. Drop spoonfuls of the mixture onto a baking sheet lined with parchment paper.
5. Flatten each cookie slightly with the back of a spoon.
6. Bake for 15 minutes, or until golden brown.
7. Allow to cool before serving.

TIPS:
- Add dark chocolate chips for an extra treat.
- Store in an airtight container for up to 3 days.

N.V.: Calories: 80, Fat: 2.5g, Carbs: 14g, Protein: 2g, Sugar: 5g, Sodium: 50 mg, Potassium: 150 mg, Cholesterol: 0 mg

APPLE CINNAMON MUFFINS

PREPARATION TIME: 15 min
COOKING TIME: 25 min
MODE OF COOKING: Baking
SERVINGS: 12 muffins
INGREDIENTS:
- 2 cups whole wheat flour
- 1 cup unsweetened applesauce
- 1/2 cup honey
- 1/4 cup coconut oil, melted
- 2 large eggs
- 1 tsp vanilla extract
- 1 tsp baking soda
- 1 tsp cinnamon
- 1/2 tsp salt
- 1 apple, peeled and finely chopped

DIRECTIONS:
1. Preheat oven to 350°F (175°C). Line a muffin tin with paper liners.
2. In a large bowl, mix together flour, baking soda, cinnamon, and salt.
3. In another bowl, whisk together applesauce, honey, coconut oil, eggs, and vanilla extract.
4. Combine wet and dry ingredients, then fold in the chopped apple.
5. Divide the batter evenly among the muffin cups.
6. Bake for 25 minutes, or until a toothpick inserted into the center comes out clean.
7. Allow to cool before serving.

TIPS:
- Add walnuts or pecans for added texture.
- Substitute honey with maple syrup for a different flavor.

N.V.: Calories: 150, Fat: 6g, Carbs: 22g, Protein: 3g, Sugar: 12g, Sodium: 150 mg, Potassium: 100 mg, Cholesterol: 25 mg

COCONUT DATE BALLS

PREPARATION TIME: 10 min
COOKING TIME: N/A
MODE OF COOKING: N/A
SERVINGS: 15 balls
INGREDIENTS:
- 1 cup Medjool dates, pitted
- 1 cup unsweetened shredded coconut
- 1/2 cup almonds
- 1 Tbsp coconut oil
- 1 tsp vanilla extract
- 1/4 tsp salt

DIRECTIONS:
1. In a food processor, combine dates, 1/2 cup shredded coconut, almonds, coconut oil, vanilla extract, and salt. Process until mixture is well combined and sticky.
2. Roll the mixture into 1-inch balls.
3. Roll each ball in the remaining shredded coconut to coat.
4. Refrigerate for at least 30 minutes before serving.

TIPS:
- Add cocoa powder for a chocolatey twist.
- Store in an airtight container in the fridge for up to a week.

N.V.: Calories: 90, Fat: 6g, Carbs: 12g, Protein: 1g, Sugar: 9g, Sodium: 20 mg, Potassium: 150 mg, Cholesterol: 0 mg

BERRY YOGURT POPSICLES

PREPARATION TIME: 10 min
COOKING TIME: N/A (Freeze for 4 hours)
MODE OF COOKING: Freezing
SERVINGS: 6 popsicles
INGREDIENTS:
- 2 cups Greek yogurt
- 1 cup mixed berries (strawberries, blueberries, raspberries)
- 1/4 cup honey
- 1 tsp vanilla extract

DIRECTIONS:
1. In a blender, combine Greek yogurt, mixed berries, honey, and vanilla extract. Blend until smooth.
2. Pour the mixture into popsicle molds.
3. Insert sticks and freeze for at least 4 hours, or until solid.
4. To release popsicles, run warm water over the outside of the molds for a few seconds.

TIPS:
- Use different fruits for variety.
- Add a splash of lemon juice for a tangy flavor.

N.V.: Calories: 100, Fat: 2g, Carbs: 16g, Protein: 6g, Sugar: 14g, Sodium: 30 mg, Potassium: 150 mg, Cholesterol: 5 mg

CHOCOLATE AVOCADO MOUSSE

PREPARATION TIME: 10 min
COOKING TIME: N/A
MODE OF COOKING: N/A
SERVINGS: 4
INGREDIENTS:
- 2 ripe avocados
- 1/4 cup cocoa powder
- 1/4 cup honey
- 1/4 cup almond milk
- 1 tsp vanilla extract
- A pinch of salt

DIRECTIONS:
1. In a blender, combine avocados, cocoa powder, honey, almond milk, vanilla extract, and salt. Blend until smooth and creamy.
2. Spoon the mousse into serving bowls.
3. Refrigerate for at least 30 minutes before serving.

TIPS:
- Top with fresh berries or a sprinkle of nuts.
- Adjust sweetness by adding more or less honey.

N.V.: Calories: 200, Fat: 14g, Carbs: 22g, Protein: 2g, Sugar: 15g, Sodium: 60 mg, Potassium: 500 mg, Cholesterol: 0 mg

BLUEBERRY OAT MUFFINS

PREPARATION TIME: 10 min
COOKING TIME: 20 min
MODE OF COOKING: Baking
SERVINGS: 12 muffins
INGREDIENTS:

- 1 cup whole wheat flour
- 1 cup rolled oats
- 1/2 cup applesauce
- 1/2 cup honey
- 1/2 cup skim milk
- 1 large egg
- 1 tsp vanilla extract
- 1 tsp baking powder
- 1/2 tsp baking soda
- 1/4 tsp salt
- 1 cup fresh blueberries

DIRECTIONS:

1. Preheat oven to 350°F (175°C). Line a muffin tin with paper liners.
2. In a large bowl, mix together flour, oats, baking powder, baking soda, and salt.
3. In another bowl, whisk together applesauce, honey, skim milk, egg, and vanilla extract.
4. Combine wet and dry ingredients, then gently fold in the blueberries.
5. Divide the batter evenly among the muffin cups.
6. Bake for 20 minutes, or until a toothpick inserted into the center comes out clean.
7. Allow to cool before serving.

TIPS:

- Substitute blueberries with raspberries or blackberries.
- Add a sprinkle of cinnamon for extra flavor.

N.V.: Calories: 120, Fat: 1.5g, Carbs: 26g, Protein: 3g, Sugar: 12g, Sodium: 100 mg, Potassium: 70 mg, Cholesterol: 15 mg

PUMPKIN SPICE BREAD

PREPARATION TIME: 15 min
COOKING TIME: 50 min
MODE OF COOKING: Baking
SERVINGS: 12 slices
INGREDIENTS:

- 1 3/4 cups whole wheat flour
- 1 cup canned pumpkin
- 1/2 cup honey
- 1/2 cup unsweetened applesauce
- 2 large eggs
- 1 tsp vanilla extract
- 1 tsp baking soda
- 1/2 tsp baking powder
- 1/2 tsp salt
- 1 tsp ground cinnamon
- 1/2 tsp ground nutmeg
- 1/4 tsp ground ginger
- 1/4 tsp ground cloves

DIRECTIONS:

1. Preheat oven to 350°F (175°C). Grease a loaf pan.
2. In a large bowl, mix together flour, baking soda, baking powder, salt, cinnamon, nutmeg, ginger, and cloves.
3. In another bowl, whisk together pumpkin, honey, applesauce, eggs, and vanilla extract.
4. Combine wet and dry ingredients, stirring until just combined.
5. Pour batter into the prepared loaf pan.
6. Bake for 50 minutes, or until a toothpick inserted into the center comes out clean.
7. Allow to cool before slicing and serving.

TIPS:

- Add chopped nuts or raisins for added texture.
- Serve with a dollop of Greek yogurt for extra protein.

N.V.: Calories: 130, Fat: 2g, Carbs: 26g, Protein: 3g, Sugar: 12g, Sodium: 160 mg, Potassium: 100 mg, Cholesterol: 30 mg

LEMON POPPY SEED COOKIES

PREPARATION TIME: 10 min
COOKING TIME: 12 min
MODE OF COOKING: Baking
SERVINGS: 24 cookies
INGREDIENTS:
- 1 cup whole wheat flour
- 1/2 cup oat flour
- 1/2 cup honey
- 1/4 cup unsweetened applesauce
- 2 large egg whites
- 2 Tbsp poppy seeds
- 1 tsp lemon zest
- 1/2 tsp baking soda
- 1/4 tsp salt
- 1/2 tsp vanilla extract

DIRECTIONS:
1. Preheat oven to 350°F (175°C). Line a baking sheet with parchment paper.
2. In a large bowl, mix together whole wheat flour, oat flour, poppy seeds, lemon zest, baking soda, and salt.
3. In another bowl, whisk together honey, applesauce, egg whites, and vanilla extract.
4. Combine wet and dry ingredients, stirring until just combined.
5. Drop spoonfuls of dough onto the prepared baking sheet.
6. Bake for 10-12 minutes, or until edges are golden brown.
7. Allow to cool before serving.

TIPS:
- Use orange zest instead of lemon for a different flavor.
- Store in an airtight container for up to 3 days.

N.V.: Calories: 60, Fat: 1g, Carbs: 12g, Protein: 2g, Sugar: 7g, Sodium: 50 mg, Potassium: 30 mg, Cholesterol: 0 mg

CARROT CAKE BARS

PREPARATION TIME: 15 min
COOKING TIME: 25 min
MODE OF COOKING: Baking
SERVINGS: 16 bars
INGREDIENTS:
- 1 1/2 cups whole wheat flour
- 1/2 cup oat flour
- 1/2 cup honey
- 1/2 cup unsweetened applesauce
- 2 large eggs
- 1 tsp vanilla extract
- 1 tsp baking soda
- 1/2 tsp baking powder
- 1/2 tsp salt
- 1 tsp ground cinnamon
- 1/2 tsp ground nutmeg
- 1/4 tsp ground ginger
- 1 cup grated carrots
- 1/2 cup raisins

DIRECTIONS:
1. Preheat oven to 350°F (175°C). Grease a 9x9-inch baking pan.
2. In a large bowl, mix together whole wheat flour, oat flour, baking soda, baking powder, salt, cinnamon, nutmeg, and ginger.
3. In another bowl, whisk together honey, applesauce, eggs, and vanilla extract.
4. Combine wet and dry ingredients, then fold in the grated carrots and raisins.
5. Pour batter into the prepared baking pan.
6. Bake for 25 minutes, or until a toothpick inserted into the center comes out clean.
7. Allow to cool before cutting into bars and serving.

TIPS:
- Add chopped nuts for added texture.
- Top with a light cream cheese frosting for extra sweetness.

N.V.: Calories: 120, Fat: 2g, Carbs: 24g, Protein: 3g, Sugar: 12g, Sodium: 100 mg, Potassium: 120 mg, Cholesterol: 30 mg

BANANA BREAD WITH WALNUTS

PREPARATION TIME: 10 min
COOKING TIME: 50 min
MODE OF COOKING: Baking
SERVINGS: 12 slices
INGREDIENTS:
- 1 1/2 cups whole wheat flour
- 1/2 cup oat flour
- 1/2 cup honey
- 1/4 cup unsweetened applesauce
- 2 large eggs
- 1/4 cup skim milk
- 1 tsp vanilla extract
- 1 tsp baking soda
- 1/2 tsp salt
- 3 ripe bananas, mashed
- 1/2 cup chopped walnuts

DIRECTIONS:
1. Preheat oven to 350°F (175°C). Grease a loaf pan.
2. In a large bowl, mix together whole wheat flour, oat flour, baking soda, and salt.
3. In another bowl, whisk together honey, applesauce, eggs, skim milk, and vanilla extract.
4. Combine wet and dry ingredients, then fold in the mashed bananas and chopped walnuts.
5. Pour batter into the prepared loaf pan.
6. Bake for 50 minutes, or until a toothpick inserted into the center comes out clean.
7. Allow to cool before slicing and serving.

TIPS:
- Add a handful of chocolate chips for extra sweetness.
- Use pecans instead of walnuts for a different flavor.

N.V.: Calories: 150, Fat: 4g, Carbs: 26g, Protein: 3g, Sugar: 14g, Sodium: 150 mg, Potassium: 200 mg, Cholesterol: 30 mg

•7.3 FRUIT-FOCUSED SWEETS: FRESH IDEAS FOR DESSERT THAT ARE EASY ON THE STOMACH.

BERRY TART WITH ALMOND CRUST

PREPARATION TIME: 15 min
COOKING TIME: 15 min
MODE OF COOKING: Baking
SERVINGS: 8
INGREDIENTS:
- **Crust:**
  - 1 cup almond flour
  - 2 Tbsp coconut oil, melted
  - 2 Tbsp honey
  - 1/4 tsp salt
- **Filling:**
  - 1 cup Greek yogurt
  - 2 Tbsp honey
  - 1 tsp vanilla extract
- **Topping:**
  - 1 cup mixed berries (strawberries, blueberries, raspberries)

DIRECTIONS:
1. Preheat oven to 350°F (175°C).
2. In a bowl, mix almond flour, melted coconut oil, honey, and salt until combined.
3. Press the mixture into the bottom of a tart pan.
4. Bake for 10-15 minutes until the crust is golden brown. Let it cool completely.
5. In a separate bowl, mix Greek yogurt, honey, and vanilla extract until smooth.
6. Spread the yogurt mixture evenly over the cooled crust.
7. Top with mixed berries.
8. Serve immediately or refrigerate until ready to serve.

TIPS:
- Use a variety of berries for a colorful and flavorful tart.
- Add a sprinkle of lemon zest for a fresh finish.

N.V.: Calories: 150, Fat: 10g, Carbs: 12g, Protein: 4g, Sugar: 8g, Sodium: 50 mg, Potassium: 100 mg, Cholesterol: 0 mg

BAKED PEACHES WITH HONEY AND ALMONDS

PREPARATION TIME: 5 min
COOKING TIME: 20 min
MODE OF COOKING: Baking
SERVINGS: 4
INGREDIENTS:

- 4 ripe peaches, halved and pitted
- 2 Tbsp honey
- 1/4 cup sliced almonds
- 1/2 tsp cinnamon

DIRECTIONS:

1. Preheat oven to 375°F (190°C).
2. Place peach halves in a baking dish, cut side up.
3. Drizzle each peach half with honey and sprinkle with sliced almonds and cinnamon.
4. Bake for 20 minutes or until peaches are tender.
5. Serve warm.

TIPS:

- Serve with a dollop of Greek yogurt or a scoop of vanilla ice cream.
- Substitute peaches with nectarines or plums.

N.V.: Calories: 120, Fat: 4g, Carbs: 21g, Protein: 2g, Sugar: 18g, Sodium: 0 mg, Potassium: 250 mg, Cholesterol: 0 mg

MANGO SORBET

PREPARATION TIME: 10 min
COOKING TIME: N/A (Freeze for 4 hours)
MODE OF COOKING: Freezing
SERVINGS: 4
INGREDIENTS:

- 3 ripe mangoes, peeled and cubed
- 1/4 cup honey
- 1/4 cup lime juice
- 1/2 cup water

DIRECTIONS:

1. In a blender, combine mangoes, honey, lime juice, and water. Blend until smooth.
2. Pour the mixture into a freezer-safe container.
3. Freeze for at least 4 hours or until firm.
4. Scoop and serve.

TIPS:

- Add a few mint leaves for a refreshing twist.
- Use an ice cream maker for a smoother texture.

N.V.: Calories: 130, Fat: 0g, Carbs: 34g, Protein: 1g, Sugar: 29g, Sodium: 5 mg, Potassium: 300 mg, Cholesterol: 0 mg

STRAWBERRY BANANA SMOOTHIE BOWL

PREPARATION TIME: 5 min
COOKING TIME: N/A
MODE OF COOKING: Blending
SERVINGS: 2
INGREDIENTS:

- 1 banana, sliced and frozen
- 1 cup strawberries, hulled and frozen
- 1/2 cup Greek yogurt
- 1/2 cup almond milk
- 1 Tbsp honey
- Toppings: granola, sliced almonds, fresh berries, chia seeds

DIRECTIONS:

1. In a blender, combine frozen banana, frozen strawberries, Greek yogurt, almond milk, and honey. Blend until smooth and thick.
2. Pour the smoothie into bowls.
3. Top with granola, sliced almonds, fresh berries, and chia seeds.
4. Serve immediately.

TIPS:

- Use different frozen fruits for variety.
- Add a scoop of protein powder for an extra boost.

N.V.: Calories: 220, Fat: 6g, Carbs: 38g, Protein: 8g, Sugar: 24g, Sodium: 50 mg, Potassium: 450 mg, Cholesterol: 5 mg

PINEAPPLE COCONUT BARS

PREPARATION TIME: 15 min
COOKING TIME: 30 min
MODE OF COOKING: Baking
SERVINGS: 12 bars
INGREDIENTS:
- **Crust:**
    - 1 cup whole wheat flour
    - 1/2 cup shredded coconut
    - 1/4 cup honey
    - 1/4 cup coconut oil, melted
    - 1/4 tsp salt
- **Filling:**
    - 2 cups fresh pineapple, diced
    - 2 Tbsp cornstarch
    - 1 Tbsp lemon juice
    - 1 Tbsp honey

DIRECTIONS:
1. Preheat oven to 350°F (175°C). Grease a 9x9-inch baking pan.
2. In a bowl, mix flour, shredded coconut, honey, melted coconut oil, and salt until combined.
3. Press the mixture into the bottom of the prepared baking pan.
4. Bake for 10 minutes or until lightly golden.
5. In another bowl, combine diced pineapple, cornstarch, lemon juice, and honey.
6. Spread the pineapple mixture over the baked crust.
7. Bake for an additional 20 minutes or until the filling is set.
8. Allow to cool before cutting into bars.

TIPS:
- Use canned pineapple if fresh is not available.
- Add a sprinkle of toasted coconut on top for extra flavor.

N.V.: Calories: 140, Fat: 6g, Carbs: 22g, Protein: 2g, Sugar: 12g, Sodium: 50 mg, Potassium: 100 mg, Cholesterol: 0 mg

CHAPTER 8: DRINKS FOR DIGESTIVE HEALTH

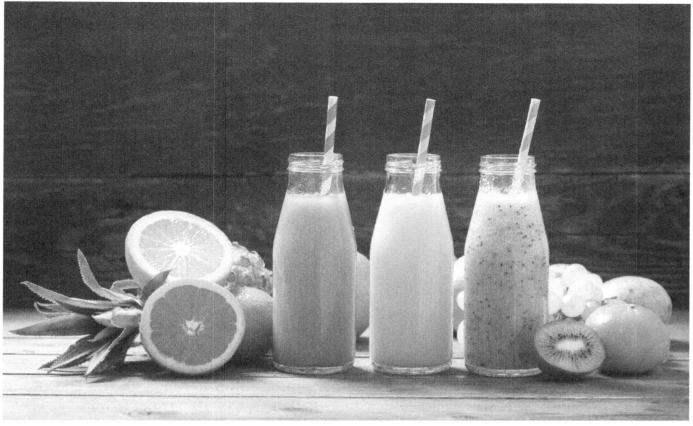

As we navigate the intricacies of our daily lives, it becomes clear that what we drink is just as important as what we eat. The right beverages can soothe, rejuvenate, and invigorate, playing a crucial role in our overall well-being. Drinks tailored for digestive health can be a transformative addition to our routines, offering not just hydration but also a blend of ingredients that promote a balanced and harmonious digestive system.

Imagine starting your day with a warm cup of ginger tea, its spicy aroma gently waking your senses and preparing your digestive tract for the meals ahead. Or consider a mid-afternoon break with a refreshing green smoothie, packed with leafy greens, fruits, and probiotics that work together to support your gut health. These drinks are more than just thirst quenchers—they are daily rituals that nurture and heal from within.

In this chapter, we explore a variety of beverages designed to support and enhance digestive health. Each recipe is crafted with care, focusing on ingredients known for their soothing and healing properties. From herbal teas that calm and cleanse to nutrient-dense smoothies that provide a burst of energy, these drinks are your companions in the journey towards better digestive wellness.

You'll find herbal infusions that have been cherished for centuries, like chamomile and peppermint, each sip offering relief from digestive discomfort and promoting relaxation. These teas are perfect for winding down in the evening or providing a gentle start to your day. We also delve into the world of fermented drinks like kefir and kombucha, whose probiotics are celebrated for their ability to balance gut flora and improve digestion.

Nutrient-dense smoothies make an appearance too, combining the goodness of fruits, vegetables, and seeds into vibrant blends that are as tasty as they are beneficial. Imagine a smoothie where the sweetness of mangoes meets the earthiness of spinach, all brought together with a splash of coconut water a drink that not only delights the palate but also nourishes the body.

As you explore these recipes, you'll discover that drinks for digestive health can be both delicious and functional. They are simple yet effective ways to support your body's natural processes, helping you feel your best every day. So, raise your glass to better digestion and overall health, one sip at a time.

•8.1 BEVERAGES THAT AID DIGESTION: HYDRATING WITH A PURPOSE.

GINGER MINT LEMONADE

PREPARATION TIME: 10 min
COOKING TIME: N/A
MODE OF COOKING: N/A
SERVINGS: 4
INGREDIENTS:
- 4 cups water
- 1/4 cup fresh lemon juice
- 1/4 cup honey
- 2 Tbsp fresh ginger, grated
- 1/4 cup fresh mint leaves
- Lemon slices for garnish
- Mint sprigs for garnish

DIRECTIONS:
1. In a large pitcher, combine water, fresh lemon juice, honey, and grated ginger.
2. Stir well until the honey is dissolved.
3. Add fresh mint leaves and stir again.
4. Chill in the refrigerator for at least 30 minutes.
5. Serve over ice, garnished with lemon slices and mint sprigs.

TIPS:
- Use sparkling water for a fizzy version.
- Add a pinch of turmeric for additional health benefits.

N.V.: Calories: 40, Fat: 0g, Carbs: 11g, Protein: 0g, Sugar: 10g, Sodium: 5 mg, Potassium: 40 mg, Cholesterol: 0 mg

ALOE VERA GREEN JUICE

PREPARATION TIME: 10 min
COOKING TIME: N/A
MODE OF COOKING: Blending
SERVINGS: 2
INGREDIENTS:
- 1 cup aloe vera gel
- 1 cup spinach
- 1/2 cucumber, chopped
- 1 green apple, chopped
- 1 Tbsp fresh lemon juice
- 1 cup coconut water

DIRECTIONS:
1. In a blender, combine aloe vera gel, spinach, cucumber, green apple, lemon juice, and coconut water.
2. Blend until smooth.
3. Pour into glasses and serve immediately.

TIPS:
- Add a small piece of ginger for extra zing.
- Use frozen spinach for a colder, thicker drink.

N.V.: Calories: 60, Fat: 0g, Carbs: 15g, Protein: 1g, Sugar: 10g, Sodium: 30 mg, Potassium: 200 mg, Cholesterol: 0 mg

FENNEL AND APPLE DETOX DRINK

PREPARATION TIME: 10 min
COOKING TIME: N/A
MODE OF COOKING: Blending
SERVINGS: 2
INGREDIENTS:
- 1 fennel bulb, chopped
- 1 green apple, chopped
- 1/2 cucumber, chopped
- 1 Tbsp fresh lemon juice
- 1 cup cold water

DIRECTIONS:
1. In a blender, combine fennel, green apple, cucumber, lemon juice, and cold water.
2. Blend until smooth.
3. Pour into glasses and serve immediately.

TIPS:
- Garnish with fennel fronds for extra flavor.
- Use chilled ingredients for a refreshing drink.

N.V.: Calories: 45, Fat: 0g, Carbs: 11g, Protein: 1g, Sugar: 7g, Sodium: 20 mg, Potassium: 150 mg, Cholesterol: 0 mg

TURMERIC GINGER TEA

PREPARATION TIME: 5 min
COOKING TIME: 5 min
MODE OF COOKING: Boiling
SERVINGS: 2
INGREDIENTS:

- 2 cups water
- 1 tsp fresh ginger, grated
- 1 tsp ground turmeric
- 1 Tbsp honey
- 1 Tbsp fresh lemon juice
- Black pepper, to taste

DIRECTIONS:

1. In a small saucepan, bring water to a boil.
2. Add grated ginger and ground turmeric. Reduce heat and simmer for 5 minutes.
3. Remove from heat and stir in honey and lemon juice.
4. Pour into mugs and add a pinch of black pepper.
5. Serve warm.

TIPS:

- Add a cinnamon stick while simmering for added flavor.
- Strain the tea before serving if desired.

N.V.: Calories: 30, Fat: 0g, Carbs: 8g, Protein: 0g, Sugar: 7g, Sodium: 5 mg, Potassium: 50 mg, Cholesterol: 0 mg

PINEAPPLE MINT SMOOTHIE

PREPARATION TIME: 5 min
COOKING TIME: N/A
MODE OF COOKING: Blending
SERVINGS: 2
INGREDIENTS:

- 1 cup fresh pineapple, chopped
- 1/2 cup Greek yogurt
- 1/2 cup coconut water
- 1 Tbsp fresh mint leaves
- 1 tsp honey
- Ice cubes (optional)

DIRECTIONS:

1. In a blender, combine pineapple, Greek yogurt, coconut water, mint leaves, and honey.
2. Blend until smooth.
3. Add ice cubes if desired and blend again.
4. Pour into glasses and serve immediately.

TIPS:

- Use frozen pineapple for a thicker smoothie.
- Add a handful of spinach for extra nutrients.

N.V.: Calories: 90, Fat: 1g, Carbs: 19g, Protein: 4g, Sugar: 15g, Sodium: 35 mg, Potassium: 200 mg, Cholesterol: 2 mg

•8.2 NUTRIENT-DENSE SMOOTHIES: BLENDS FOR HEALTH AND TASTE.

GREEN DETOX SMOOTHIE

PREPARATION TIME: 5 min
COOKING TIME: N/A
MODE OF COOKING: Blending
SERVINGS: 2
INGREDIENTS:

- 1 cup spinach
- 1/2 cucumber, chopped
- 1 green apple, chopped
- 1/2 avocado
- 1 cup coconut water
- 1 Tbsp fresh lemon juice
- 1 tsp honey
- Ice cubes (optional)

DIRECTIONS:

1. In a blender, combine spinach, cucumber, green apple, avocado, coconut water, lemon juice, and honey.
2. Blend until smooth.
3. Add ice cubes if desired and blend again.
4. Pour into glasses and serve immediately.

TIPS:

- Add a small piece of ginger for a spicy kick.
- Use frozen spinach for a thicker texture.

N.V.: Calories: 160, Fat: 8g, Carbs: 21g, Protein: 3g, Sugar: 12g, Sodium: 45 mg, Potassium: 500 mg, Cholesterol: 0 mg

BERRY PROTEIN SMOOTHIE

PREPARATION TIME: 5 min
COOKING TIME: N/A
MODE OF COOKING: Blending
SERVINGS: 2
INGREDIENTS:
- 1 cup mixed berries (strawberries, blueberries, raspberries)
- 1 banana
- 1/2 cup Greek yogurt
- 1 cup almond milk
- 1 scoop vanilla protein powder
- 1 Tbsp chia seeds
- Ice cubes (optional)

DIRECTIONS:
1. In a blender, combine mixed berries, banana, Greek yogurt, almond milk, protein powder, and chia seeds.
2. Blend until smooth.
3. Add ice cubes if desired and blend again.
4. Pour into glasses and serve immediately.

TIPS:
- Use a variety of berries for a richer flavor.
- Add a handful of spinach for extra nutrients.

N.V.: Calories: 250, Fat: 4g, Carbs: 35g, Protein: 20g, Sugar: 20g, Sodium: 80 mg, Potassium: 600 mg, Cholesterol: 5 mg

TROPICAL TURMERIC SMOOTHIE

PREPARATION TIME: 5 min
COOKING TIME: N/A
MODE OF COOKING: Blending
SERVINGS: 2
INGREDIENTS:
- 1 cup pineapple chunks
- 1 mango, peeled and chopped
- 1 banana
- 1 cup coconut milk
- 1 tsp ground turmeric
- 1/2 tsp ginger powder
- Ice cubes (optional)

DIRECTIONS:
1. In a blender, combine pineapple, mango, banana, coconut milk, turmeric, and ginger powder.
2. Blend until smooth.
3. Add ice cubes if desired and blend again.
4. Pour into glasses and serve immediately.

TIPS:
- Garnish with a sprinkle of coconut flakes.
- Use fresh ginger for a stronger flavor.

N.V.: Calories: 220, Fat: 7g, Carbs: 42g, Protein: 2g, Sugar: 30g, Sodium: 20 mg, Potassium: 600 mg, Cholesterol: 0 mg

CHOCOLATE ALMOND BUTTER SMOOTHIE

PREPARATION TIME: 5 min
COOKING TIME: N/A
MODE OF COOKING: Blending
SERVINGS: 2
INGREDIENTS:
- 1 banana
- 2 Tbsp almond butter
- 1 cup almond milk
- 1 Tbsp cocoa powder
- 1 tsp honey
- 1/2 tsp vanilla extract
- Ice cubes (optional)

DIRECTIONS:
1. In a blender, combine banana, almond butter, almond milk, cocoa powder, honey, and vanilla extract.
2. Blend until smooth.
3. Add ice cubes if desired and blend again.
4. Pour into glasses and serve immediately.

TIPS:
- Add a scoop of protein powder for extra protein.
- Garnish with a sprinkle of cocoa nibs or almond slices.

N.V.: Calories: 210, Fat: 12g, Carbs: 23g, Protein: 5g, Sugar: 15g, Sodium: 100 mg, Potassium: 400 mg, Cholesterol: 0 mg

AVOCADO PINEAPPLE SMOOTHIE

PREPARATION TIME: 5 min
COOKING TIME: N/A
MODE OF COOKING: Blending
SERVINGS: 2
INGREDIENTS:

- 1 ripe avocado
- 1 cup pineapple chunks
- 1 cup spinach
- 1 cup coconut water
- 1 Tbsp lime juice
- Ice cubes (optional)

DIRECTIONS:

1. In a blender, combine avocado, pineapple, spinach, coconut water, and lime juice.
2. Blend until smooth.
3. Add ice cubes if desired and blend again.
4. Pour into glasses and serve immediately.

TIPS:

- Add a small piece of ginger for a refreshing twist.
- Use frozen pineapple for a thicker consistency.

N.V.: Calories: 180, Fat: 10g, Carbs: 25g, Protein: 2g, Sugar: 15g, Sodium: 30 mg, Potassium: 500 mg, Cholesterol: 0 mg

•8.3 HERBAL TEAS: SOOTHING RECIPES FOR DIGESTIVE EASE.

CHAMOMILE GINGER TEA

PREPARATION TIME: 5 min
COOKING TIME: 10 min
MODE OF COOKING: Steeping
SERVINGS: 2
INGREDIENTS:

- 2 cups water
- 2 chamomile tea bags
- 1-inch piece fresh ginger, sliced
- 1 Tbsp honey
- Lemon slices for garnish

DIRECTIONS:

1. Bring water to a boil in a small saucepan.
2. Add the sliced ginger and boil for 5 minutes.
3. Remove from heat and add chamomile tea bags. Let steep for 5 minutes.
4. Remove tea bags and ginger slices.
5. Stir in honey.
6. Pour into cups and garnish with lemon slices.

TIPS:

- Use fresh chamomile flowers if available.
- Add a sprig of mint for extra freshness.

N.V.: Calories: 30, Fat: 0g, Carbs: 8g, Protein: 0g, Sugar: 7g, Sodium: 5 mg, Potassium: 10 mg, Cholesterol: 0 mg

PEPPERMINT FENNEL TEA

PREPARATION TIME: 5 min
COOKING TIME: 10 min
MODE OF COOKING: Steeping
SERVINGS: 2
INGREDIENTS:

- 2 cups water
- 2 tsp dried peppermint leaves
- 1 tsp fennel seeds
- 1 Tbsp honey
- Fresh mint leaves for garnish

DIRECTIONS:

1. Bring water to a boil in a small saucepan.
2. Add dried peppermint leaves and fennel seeds.
3. Remove from heat and let steep for 10 minutes.
4. Strain the tea into cups.
5. Stir in honey.
6. Garnish with fresh mint leaves.

TIPS:

- Use fresh peppermint leaves for a stronger flavor.
- Add a squeeze of lemon for a citrus twist.

N.V.: Calories: 25, Fat: 0g, Carbs: 7g, Protein: 0g, Sugar: 7g, Sodium: 5 mg, Potassium: 10 mg, Cholesterol: 0 mg

LEMON BALM AND LICORICE ROOT TEA

PREPARATION TIME: 5 min
COOKING TIME: 10 min
MODE OF COOKING: Steeping
SERVINGS: 2
INGREDIENTS:

- 2 cups water
- 2 tsp dried lemon balm
- 1 tsp dried licorice root
- 1 Tbsp honey
- Lemon slices for garnish

DIRECTIONS:

1. Bring water to a boil in a small saucepan.
2. Add dried lemon balm and dried licorice root.
3. Remove from heat and let steep for 10 minutes.
4. Strain the tea into cups.
5. Stir in honey.
6. Garnish with lemon slices.

TIPS:

- Use fresh lemon balm for a more vibrant flavor.
- Add a pinch of dried lavender for a soothing aroma.

N.V.: Calories: 25, Fat: 0g, Carbs: 7g, Protein: 0g, Sugar: 7g, Sodium: 5 mg, Potassium: 10 mg, Cholesterol: 0 mg

CINNAMON CLOVE TEA

PREPARATION TIME: 5 min
COOKING TIME: 10 min
MODE OF COOKING: Steeping
SERVINGS: 2
INGREDIENTS:

- 2 cups water
- 1 cinnamon stick
- 4 whole cloves
- 1 Tbsp honey
- Orange slices for garnish

DIRECTIONS:

1. Bring water to a boil in a small saucepan.
2. Add cinnamon stick and whole cloves.
3. Remove from heat and let steep for 10 minutes.
4. Strain the tea into cups.
5. Stir in honey.
6. Garnish with orange slices.

TIPS:

- Add a star anise for a more complex flavor.
- Serve with a cinnamon stick in the cup for extra spice.

N.V.: Calories: 30, Fat: 0g, Carbs: 8g, Protein: 0g, Sugar: 7g, Sodium: 5 mg, Potassium: 10 mg, Cholesterol: 0 mg

ROSEMARY AND LAVENDER TEA

PREPARATION TIME: 5 min
COOKING TIME: 10 min
MODE OF COOKING: Steeping
SERVINGS: 2
INGREDIENTS:

- 2 cups water
- 1 tsp dried rosemary
- 1 tsp dried lavender flowers
- 1 Tbsp honey
- Fresh rosemary sprigs for garnish

DIRECTIONS:

1. Bring water to a boil in a small saucepan.
2. Add dried rosemary and dried lavender flowers.
3. Remove from heat and let steep for 10 minutes.
4. Strain the tea into cups.
5. Stir in honey.
6. Garnish with fresh rosemary sprigs.

TIPS:

- Use fresh rosemary and lavender for a more aromatic tea.
- Add a slice of lemon for a citrusy note.

N.V.: Calories: 25, Fat: 0g, Carbs: 7g, Protein: 0g, Sugar: 7g, Sodium: 5 mg, Potassium: 10 mg, Cholesterol: 0 mg

CHAPTER 9: FESTIVE FOODS AND CELEBRATIONS

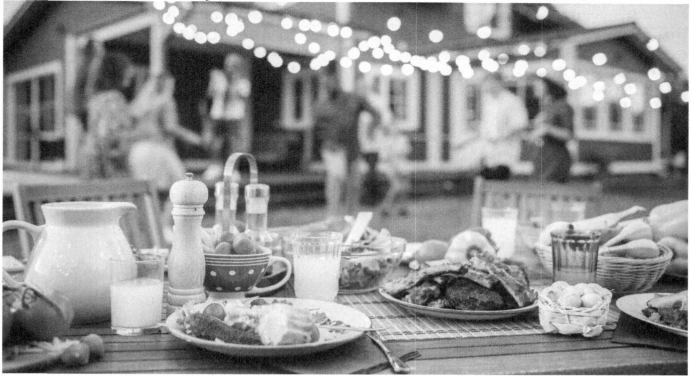

There's a certain magic that comes with festive occasions and celebrations. These moments, filled with laughter, joy, and togetherness, often revolve around a central element: food. The dishes we share during these times become more than just meals; they turn into cherished memories, linking us to the people and moments we hold dear. Whether it's a grand holiday feast or an intimate gathering, the right food can elevate the spirit of any celebration.

Imagine a table adorned with vibrant, colorful dishes, each one carefully prepared and beautifully presented. The aroma of freshly baked bread, the sizzle of a roasting turkey, and the sweet scent of a spiced dessert waft through the air, creating an atmosphere of warmth and anticipation. These are the moments where food transcends its basic function of nourishment and becomes a language of love, hospitality, and joy.

In this chapter, we embark on a culinary journey through festive foods and celebrations, exploring recipes that are designed to delight and impress. Each dish is crafted with the idea of bringing people together, celebrating the essence of the occasion, and ensuring that everyone leaves the table with a smile. From appetizers that tantalize the taste buds to main courses that serve as the centerpiece of the meal, these recipes are your guide to creating unforgettable culinary experiences.

You'll find inspiration in dishes that are both traditional and innovative, each one offering a unique twist on festive favorites. Picture a succulent roast, perfectly seasoned and cooked to perfection, served with a medley of roasted vegetables. Or imagine a dessert table laden with an array of treats, from decadent chocolate cakes to delicate fruit tarts, each one more tempting than the last.

The joy of these recipes lies not just in their taste, but in their ability to bring people together. They are designed to be shared, to spark conversations, and to create lasting memories. As you explore this chapter, you'll discover that the true essence of festive foods is their power to turn any gathering into a celebration.

So, whether you're planning a big holiday bash or a simple dinner party with friends, let these recipes inspire you to create dishes that are as festive as the occasions they celebrate. Embrace the joy of cooking, the pleasure of sharing, and the magic of making every celebration a culinary triumph.

STUFFED MINI BELL PEPPERS

PREPARATION TIME: 15 min
COOKING TIME: 10 min
MODE OF COOKING: Baking
SERVINGS: 4
INGREDIENTS:

- 12 mini bell peppers
- 1 cup cooked quinoa
- 1/2 cup feta cheese, crumbled
- 1/4 cup sun-dried tomatoes, chopped
- 2 Tbsp fresh parsley, chopped
- 1 clove garlic, minced
- 1 Tbsp olive oil
- Salt and pepper to taste

DIRECTIONS:

1. Preheat oven to 375°F (190°C).
2. Cut the tops off the mini bell peppers and remove the seeds.
3. In a bowl, mix cooked quinoa, feta cheese, sun-dried tomatoes, parsley, garlic, olive oil, salt, and pepper.
4. Stuff each mini bell pepper with the quinoa mixture.
5. Place the stuffed peppers on a baking sheet and bake for 10 minutes until the peppers are tender.
6. Serve warm.

TIPS:

- Use a mix of colorful bell peppers for a vibrant presentation.
- Add a squeeze of lemon juice for extra flavor.

N.V.: Calories: 120, Fat: 6g, Carbs: 12g, Protein: 4g, Sugar: 4g, Sodium: 150 mg, Potassium: 200 mg, Cholesterol: 10 mg

CUCUMBER AVOCADO BITES

PREPARATION TIME: 10 min
COOKING TIME: N/A
MODE OF COOKING: N/A
SERVINGS: 4
INGREDIENTS:

- 1 large cucumber
- 1 ripe avocado
- 1 Tbsp lime juice
- 1 clove garlic, minced
- 1/4 cup cherry tomatoes, diced
- Salt and pepper to taste
- Fresh cilantro for garnish

DIRECTIONS:

1. Slice the cucumber into rounds about 1/4 inch thick.
2. In a bowl, mash the avocado with lime juice, garlic, salt, and pepper.
3. Spread the avocado mixture on each cucumber round.
4. Top with diced cherry tomatoes.
5. Garnish with fresh cilantro and serve immediately.

TIPS:

- Add a sprinkle of red pepper flakes for a spicy kick.
- Serve chilled for a refreshing appetizer.

N.V.: Calories: 80, Fat: 6g, Carbs: 7g, Protein: 1g, Sugar: 2g, Sodium: 5 mg, Potassium: 250 mg, Cholesterol: 0 mg

SPINACH ARTICHOKE DIP

PREPARATION TIME: 10 min
COOKING TIME: 20 min
MODE OF COOKING: Baking
SERVINGS: 6
INGREDIENTS:
- 1 can artichoke hearts, drained and chopped
- 1 cup fresh spinach, chopped
- 1/2 cup Greek yogurt
- 1/2 cup Parmesan cheese, grated
- 1/4 cup mozzarella cheese, shredded
- 2 cloves garlic, minced
- 1 Tbsp olive oil
- Salt and pepper to taste

DIRECTIONS:
1. Preheat oven to 375°F (190°C).
2. In a bowl, mix together artichoke hearts, spinach, Greek yogurt, Parmesan cheese, mozzarella cheese, garlic, olive oil, salt, and pepper.
3. Transfer the mixture to a baking dish.
4. Bake for 20 minutes until bubbly and golden on top.
5. Serve warm with whole-grain crackers or vegetable sticks.

TIPS:
- Add a pinch of red pepper flakes for a bit of heat.
- Use frozen spinach if fresh is not available; just thaw and squeeze out excess water.

N.V.: Calories: 110, Fat: 7g, Carbs: 5g, Protein: 7g, Sugar: 1g, Sodium: 250 mg, Potassium: 150 mg, Cholesterol: 15 mg

CAPRESE SKEWERS

PREPARATION TIME: 10 min
COOKING TIME: N/A
MODE OF COOKING: N/A
SERVINGS: 4
INGREDIENTS:
- 12 cherry tomatoes
- 12 mini mozzarella balls (bocconcini)
- Fresh basil leaves
- 2 Tbsp balsamic glaze
- 1 Tbsp olive oil
- Salt and pepper to taste

DIRECTIONS:
1. Thread one cherry tomato, one mini mozzarella ball, and one basil leaf onto each skewer.
2. Arrange skewers on a serving platter.
3. Drizzle with balsamic glaze and olive oil.
4. Season with salt and pepper.
5. Serve immediately.

TIPS:
- Use colorful heirloom cherry tomatoes for added visual appeal.
- Add a slice of prosciutto for a gourmet touch.

N.V.: Calories: 80, Fat: 6g, Carbs: 3g, Protein: 4g, Sugar: 1g, Sodium: 50 mg, Potassium: 100 mg, Cholesterol: 10 mg

SWEET POTATO ROUNDS WITH GOAT CHEESE

PREPARATION TIME: 10 min
COOKING TIME: 20 min
MODE OF COOKING: Baking
SERVINGS: 4
INGREDIENTS:
- 2 large sweet potatoes
- 1/4 cup goat cheese, crumbled
- 2 Tbsp honey
- 1 Tbsp fresh rosemary, chopped
- 1 Tbsp olive oil
- Salt and pepper to taste

DIRECTIONS:
1. Preheat oven to 375°F (190°C).
2. Slice sweet potatoes into 1/4-inch rounds.
3. Toss sweet potato rounds with olive oil, salt, and pepper.
4. Arrange on a baking sheet and bake for 20 minutes until tender.
5. Top each round with a bit of goat cheese, a drizzle of honey, and a sprinkle of rosemary.
6. Serve warm.

TIPS:
- Add a few crushed walnuts for extra crunch.
- Use feta cheese as an alternative to goat cheese.

N.V.: Calories: 120, Fat: 4g, Carbs: 19g, Protein: 3g, Sugar: 7g, Sodium: 70 mg, Potassium: 300 mg, Cholesterol: 5 mg

HERB-CRUSTED SALMON

PREPARATION TIME: 15 min
COOKING TIME: 20 min
MODE OF COOKING: Baking
SERVINGS: 4
INGREDIENTS:

- 4 salmon fillets
- 2 Tbsp olive oil
- 2 Tbsp Dijon mustard
- 1/2 cup panko breadcrumbs
- 1/4 cup fresh parsley, chopped
- 2 Tbsp fresh dill, chopped
- 2 cloves garlic, minced
- Salt and pepper to taste
- Lemon wedges for serving

DIRECTIONS:

1. Preheat oven to 375°F (190°C). Line a baking sheet with parchment paper.
2. In a small bowl, mix olive oil and Dijon mustard.
3. In another bowl, combine panko breadcrumbs, parsley, dill, garlic, salt, and pepper.
4. Brush the top of each salmon fillet with the mustard mixture, then press the breadcrumb mixture onto the top of each fillet.
5. Place the salmon fillets on the prepared baking sheet.
6. Bake for 15-20 minutes, until the salmon is cooked through and the crust is golden brown.
7. Serve with lemon wedges.

TIPS:

- Serve with a side of roasted vegetables or a fresh green salad.
- Use whole grain mustard for a different flavor profile.

N.V.: Calories: 320, Fat: 18g, Carbs: 8g, Protein: 32g, Sugar: 1g, Sodium: 220 mg, Potassium: 750 mg, Cholesterol: 70 mg

MEDITERRANEAN STUFFED PEPPERS

PREPARATION TIME: 20 min
COOKING TIME: 40 min
MODE OF COOKING: Baking
SERVINGS: 4
INGREDIENTS:

- 4 large bell peppers
- 1 cup quinoa, rinsed
- 2 cups vegetable broth
- 1 can chickpeas, drained and rinsed
- 1 cup cherry tomatoes, halved
- 1/2 cup Kalamata olives, sliced
- 1/4 cup red onion, diced
- 1/2 cup feta cheese, crumbled
- 2 Tbsp olive oil
- 2 cloves garlic, minced
- 1 tsp dried oregano
- Salt and pepper to taste
- Fresh basil for garnish

DIRECTIONS:

1. Preheat oven to 375°F (190°C). Cut the tops off the bell peppers and remove the seeds.
2. In a medium saucepan, bring quinoa and vegetable broth to a boil. Reduce heat and simmer for 15 minutes, or until quinoa is tender.
3. In a large bowl, combine cooked quinoa, chickpeas, cherry tomatoes, olives, red onion, feta cheese, olive oil, garlic, oregano, salt, and pepper.
4. Stuff each bell pepper with the quinoa mixture and place them in a baking dish.
5. Cover with foil and bake for 30 minutes.
6. Remove foil and bake for an additional 10 minutes.
7. Garnish with fresh basil before serving.

TIPS:

- Use a variety of colored bell peppers for a vibrant presentation.
- Serve with a side of tzatziki sauce.

N.V.: Calories: 280, Fat: 12g, Carbs: 34g, Protein: 10g, Sugar: 8g, Sodium: 480 mg, Potassium: 600 mg, Cholesterol: 10 mg

LEMON HERB CHICKEN SKEWERS

PREPARATION TIME: 15 min
COOKING TIME: 15 min
MODE OF COOKING: Grilling
SERVINGS: 4
INGREDIENTS:

- 2 lbs. chicken breast, cut into cubes
- 1/4 cup olive oil
- 1/4 cup lemon juice
- 2 Tbsp fresh parsley, chopped
- 1 Tbsp fresh thyme, chopped
- 1 Tbsp fresh rosemary, chopped
- 2 cloves garlic, minced
- Salt and pepper to taste
- Wooden skewers, soaked in water for 30 minutes

DIRECTIONS:

1. In a large bowl, mix olive oil, lemon juice, parsley, thyme, rosemary, garlic, salt, and pepper.
2. Add the chicken cubes to the bowl and toss to coat.
3. Thread the chicken onto the skewers.
4. Preheat grill to medium-high heat.
5. Grill the skewers for 10-15 minutes, turning occasionally, until the chicken is cooked through and has grill marks.
6. Serve immediately.

TIPS:

- Serve with a side of grilled vegetables or a Greek salad.
- Add a pinch of red pepper flakes to the marinade for a bit of heat.

N.V.: Calories: 290, Fat: 15g, Carbs: 3g, Protein: 35g, Sugar: 0g, Sodium: 150 mg, Potassium: 650 mg, Cholesterol: 110 mg

VEGGIE-PACKED LASAGNA

PREPARATION TIME: 30 min
COOKING TIME: 50 min
MODE OF COOKING: Baking
SERVINGS: 8
INGREDIENTS:

- 12 lasagna noodles
- 2 cups marinara sauce
- 1 cup ricotta cheese
- 1/2 cup mozzarella cheese, shredded
- 1/2 cup Parmesan cheese, grated
- 2 cups spinach, chopped
- 1 zucchini, thinly sliced
- 1 yellow squash, thinly sliced
- 1 bell pepper, chopped
- 1/2 cup red onion, diced
- 2 cloves garlic, minced
- 2 Tbsp olive oil
- Salt and pepper to taste
- Fresh basil for garnish

DIRECTIONS:

1. Preheat oven to 375°F (190°C).
2. Cook lasagna noodles according to package instructions.
3. In a large skillet, heat olive oil over medium heat. Add garlic, red onion, bell pepper, zucchini, yellow squash, and spinach. Cook until vegetables are tender. Season with salt and pepper.
4. In a bowl, mix ricotta cheese with half of the Parmesan cheese.
5. Spread a thin layer of marinara sauce in the bottom of a baking dish. Layer with noodles, ricotta mixture, cooked vegetables, and marinara sauce. Repeat layers, ending with noodles and marinara sauce.
6. Top with mozzarella cheese and the remaining Parmesan cheese.
7. Cover with foil and bake for 30 minutes. Remove foil and bake for an additional 20 minutes until the cheese is bubbly and golden.
8. Garnish with fresh basil before serving.

TIPS:

- Use whole wheat lasagna noodles for added fiber.
- Substitute ricotta with cottage cheese for a lighter option.

N.V.: Calories: 320, Fat: 12g, Carbs: 38g, Protein: 16g, Sugar: 7g, Sodium: 420 mg, Potassium: 500 mg, Cholesterol: 30 mg

SHRIMP AND AVOCADO SALAD

PREPARATION TIME: 15 min
COOKING TIME: 5 min
MODE OF COOKING: Stovetop
SERVINGS: 4
INGREDIENTS:

- 1 lb. shrimp, peeled and deveined
- 2 avocados, diced
- 1 cup cherry tomatoes, halved
- 1/4 cup red onion, diced
- 1/4 cup fresh cilantro, chopped
- 2 Tbsp olive oil
- 2 Tbsp lime juice
- 1 clove garlic, minced
- Salt and pepper to taste

DIRECTIONS:

1. In a skillet, heat 1 Tbsp olive oil over medium heat. Add shrimp and cook until pink and opaque, about 2-3 minutes per side. Remove from heat and set aside.
2. In a large bowl, combine diced avocados, cherry tomatoes, red onion, and cilantro.
3. In a small bowl, whisk together remaining olive oil, lime juice, garlic, salt, and pepper.
4. Add cooked shrimp to the large bowl and toss with the dressing.
5. Serve immediately.

TIPS:

- Serve over mixed greens for a heartier salad.
- Add a sprinkle of red pepper flakes for a bit of spice.

N.V.: Calories: 250, Fat: 15g, Carbs: 12g, Protein: 18g, Sugar: 3g, Sodium: 320 mg, Potassium: 650 mg, Cholesterol: 170 mg

•9.3 PARTY-PERFECT DESSERTS AND SNACKS: TREATS TO CELEBRATE WITHOUT DISCOMFORT.

GREEK YOGURT FRUIT TART

PREPARATION TIME: 20 min
COOKING TIME: N/A
MODE OF COOKING: No cooking
SERVINGS: 8
INGREDIENTS:

- **Crust:**
  - 1 1/2 cups graham cracker crumbs
  - 1/4 cup coconut oil, melted
  - 2 Tbsp honey
- **Filling:**
  - 2 cups Greek yogurt
  - 2 Tbsp honey
  - 1 tsp vanilla extract
- **Topping:**
  - 1 cup mixed fresh berries (strawberries, blueberries, raspberries)
  - 1 kiwi, peeled and sliced
  - Fresh mint leaves for garnish

DIRECTIONS:

1. In a bowl, combine graham cracker crumbs, melted coconut oil, and honey. Mix well.
2. Press the mixture into the bottom of a tart pan to form the crust. Chill in the refrigerator for 15 minutes.
3. In another bowl, mix Greek yogurt, honey, and vanilla extract until smooth.
4. Spread the yogurt mixture evenly over the chilled crust.
5. Arrange the mixed berries and kiwi slices on top.
6. Garnish with fresh mint leaves and serve immediately or chill until ready to serve.

TIPS:

- Use a variety of fruits for a colorful and flavorful tart.
- Add a sprinkle of granola on top for extra crunch.

N.V.: Calories: 180, Fat: 8g, Carbs: 24g, Protein: 6g, Sugar: 16g, Sodium: 60 mg, Potassium: 150 mg, Cholesterol: 0 mg

ALMOND BUTTER ENERGY BITES

PREPARATION TIME: 10 min
COOKING TIME: N/A (Chill for 30 min)
MODE OF COOKING: No cooking
SERVINGS: 16 bites
INGREDIENTS:
- 1 cup rolled oats
- 1/2 cup almond butter
- 1/4 cup honey
- 1/4 cup ground flaxseed
- 1/4 cup mini dark chocolate chips
- 1 tsp vanilla extract

DIRECTIONS:
1. In a large bowl, combine all ingredients and mix well.
2. Roll the mixture into 1-inch balls.
3. Place the energy bites on a baking sheet lined with parchment paper and chill in the refrigerator for 30 minutes.
4. Serve chilled.

TIPS:
- Substitute almond butter with peanut butter or cashew butter.
- Add a tablespoon of chia seeds for extra fiber.

N.V.: Calories: 100, Fat: 6g, Carbs: 12g, Protein: 3g, Sugar: 7g, Sodium: 20 mg, Potassium: 100 mg, Cholesterol: 0 mg

DARK CHOCOLATE-DIPPED STRAWBERRIES

PREPARATION TIME: 10 min
COOKING TIME: 5 min
MODE OF COOKING: Stovetop
SERVINGS: 12
INGREDIENTS:
- 1-pint fresh strawberries
- 1 cup dark chocolate chips
- 1 tsp coconut oil
- 1/4 cup chopped nuts (optional)

DIRECTIONS:
1. Wash and dry the strawberries, leaving the stems on.
2. In a heatproof bowl, combine dark chocolate chips and coconut oil.
3. Melt the chocolate and coconut oil over a double boiler or in the microwave, stirring until smooth.
4. Dip each strawberry into the melted chocolate, allowing excess to drip off.
5. Place the dipped strawberries on a baking sheet lined with parchment paper.
6. If desired, sprinkle chopped nuts over the chocolate before it sets.
7. Chill in the refrigerator for 15 minutes or until the chocolate is firm.

TIPS:
- Use white chocolate or milk chocolate for variety.
- Add a drizzle of melted white chocolate for decoration.

N.V.: Calories: 70, Fat: 4g, Carbs: 10g, Protein: 1g, Sugar: 8g, Sodium: 0 mg, Potassium: 120 mg, Cholesterol: 0 mg

AVOCADO CHOCOLATE MOUSSE

PREPARATION TIME: 10 min
COOKING TIME: N/A
MODE OF COOKING: No cooking
SERVINGS: 4
INGREDIENTS:
- 2 ripe avocados
- 1/4 cup cocoa powder
- 1/4 cup honey
- 1/4 cup almond milk
- 1 tsp vanilla extract
- Fresh berries for garnish

DIRECTIONS:
1. In a blender, combine avocados, cocoa powder, honey, almond milk, and vanilla extract.
2. Blend until smooth and creamy.
3. Spoon the mousse into serving bowls.
4. Garnish with fresh berries.
5. Serve immediately or chill until ready to serve.

TIPS:
- Add a pinch of sea salt for enhanced flavor.
- Top with a dollop of whipped coconut cream.

N.V.: Calories: 160, Fat: 10g, Carbs: 20g, Protein: 2g, Sugar: 15g, Sodium: 20 mg, Potassium: 450 mg, Cholesterol: 0 mg

COCONUT MACAROONS

PREPARATION TIME: 10 min
COOKING TIME: 15 min
MODE OF COOKING: Baking
SERVINGS: 20
INGREDIENTS:

- 3 cups shredded unsweetened coconut
- 1/2 cup honey
- 1/4 cup coconut flour
- 1/4 cup coconut oil, melted
- 1 tsp vanilla extract
- 2 large egg whites
- Pinch of salt

DIRECTIONS:

1. Preheat oven to 350°F (175°C). Line a baking sheet with parchment paper.
2. In a large bowl, combine shredded coconut, honey, coconut flour, melted coconut oil, vanilla extract, egg whites, and salt. Mix well.
3. Drop spoonfuls of the mixture onto the prepared baking sheet.
4. Bake for 15 minutes or until golden brown.
5. Allow to cool before serving.

TIPS:

- Dip the bottoms of the macaroons in melted dark chocolate for extra indulgence.
- Add a tablespoon of lemon zest for a citrusy twist.

N.V.: Calories: 80, Fat: 6g, Carbs: 8g, Protein: 1g, Sugar: 6g, Sodium: 20 mg, Potassium: 70 mg, Cholesterol: 0 mg

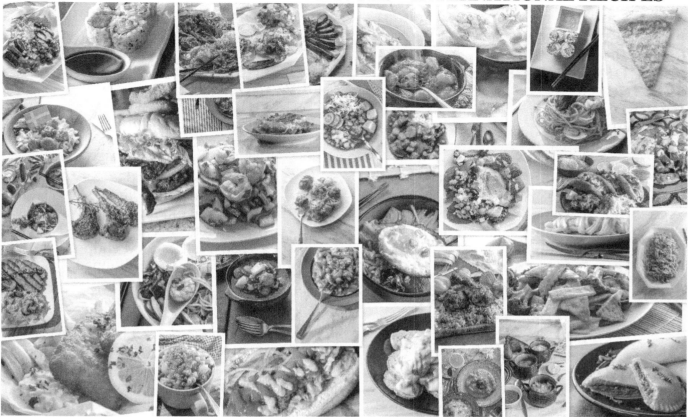

In our ever-connected world, the flavors and aromas of distant lands are just a recipe away. Culinary traditions from around the globe invite us into their kitchens, offering a taste of their culture and a glimpse into their daily lives. Cooking international recipes not only broadens our palate but also bridges cultural divides, bringing a piece of the world to our own dining tables.

Imagine the vibrant spices of India dancing on your taste buds, the comforting warmth of an Italian pasta dish, or the fresh, zesty notes of a Thai salad. Each cuisine tells a story, rich with history and tradition, and every dish becomes a journey, transporting us to far-off places and introducing us to new and exciting flavors.

In this chapter, we embark on a culinary adventure across continents, exploring recipes that capture the essence of various cultures. These international dishes are more than just meals; they are an invitation to explore, to experiment, and to appreciate the diversity that our world offers. From the robust and hearty stews of Eastern Europe to the delicate and artful sushi of Japan, this collection is designed to inspire and delight.

You'll discover recipes that are both authentic and approachable, allowing you to recreate the magic of these cuisines in your own kitchen. Picture yourself preparing a fragrant Moroccan tagine, the aromas of cinnamon and cumin filling the air, or crafting a fresh ceviche from Peru, its tangy citrus dressing perfectly balancing the tender seafood. Each recipe is a celebration of its origin, thoughtfully adapted to be enjoyed by cooks of all skill levels.

As you explore these international recipes, you'll find that cooking can be a form of travel, a way to experience the richness and variety of our world from the comfort of home. It's an opportunity to gather around the table, share stories, and create memories with flavors that are as diverse as they are delicious.

So, join us on this global gastronomic journey. Let each dish you prepare be a tribute to the world's culinary heritage, a way to honor and celebrate the multitude of tastes that make our world so wonderfully diverse. Embrace the adventure, and savor the journey with every bite.

GREEK SALAD WITH LEMON VINAIGRETTE

PREPARATION TIME: 15 min
COOKING TIME: N/A
MODE OF COOKING: No cooking
SERVINGS: 4
INGREDIENTS:

- **Salad:**
  - 1 cucumber, diced
  - 1 cup cherry tomatoes, halved
  - 1 red bell pepper, diced
  - 1/2 red onion, thinly sliced
  - 1/2 cup Kalamata olives, pitted
  - 1/4 cup feta cheese, crumbled
  - 1/4 cup fresh parsley, chopped
- **Dressing:**
  - 1/4 cup olive oil
  - 2 Tbsp fresh lemon juice
  - 1 tsp Dijon mustard
  - 1 clove garlic, minced
  - Salt and pepper to taste

DIRECTIONS:

1. In a large bowl, combine cucumber, cherry tomatoes, red bell pepper, red onion, Kalamata olives, feta cheese, and parsley.
2. In a small bowl, whisk together olive oil, lemon juice, Dijon mustard, garlic, salt, and pepper.
3. Pour the dressing over the salad and toss to combine.
4. Serve immediately.

TIPS:

- Add grilled chicken for a protein boost.
- Substitute feta cheese with goat cheese for a different flavor.

N.V.: Calories: 200, Fat: 16g, Carbs: 10g, Protein: 3g, Sugar: 5g, Sodium: 400 mg, Potassium: 400 mg, Cholesterol: 10 mg

MEDITERRANEAN QUINOA BOWL

PREPARATION TIME: 10 min
COOKING TIME: 15 min
MODE OF COOKING: Stovetop
SERVINGS: 4
INGREDIENTS:

- 1 cup quinoa, rinsed
- 2 cups vegetable broth
- 1/2 cup cherry tomatoes, halved
- 1/2 cucumber, diced
- 1/4 cup Kalamata olives, sliced
- 1/4 cup red onion, diced
- 1/4 cup feta cheese, crumbled
- 2 Tbsp fresh parsley, chopped
- 2 Tbsp fresh mint, chopped
- 1/4 cup olive oil
- 2 Tbsp fresh lemon juice
- 1 clove garlic, minced
- Salt and pepper to taste

DIRECTIONS:

1. In a medium saucepan, bring vegetable broth to a boil. Add quinoa, reduce heat, cover, and simmer for 15 minutes, or until liquid is absorbed and quinoa is tender.
2. In a large bowl, combine cooked quinoa, cherry tomatoes, cucumber, Kalamata olives, red onion, feta cheese, parsley, and mint.
3. In a small bowl, whisk together olive oil, lemon juice, garlic, salt, and pepper.
4. Pour the dressing over the quinoa mixture and toss to combine.
5. Serve warm or chilled.

TIPS:

- Add grilled shrimp or chicken for added protein.
- Use red quinoa for a colorful presentation.

N.V.: Calories: 240, Fat: 14g, Carbs: 22g, Protein: 6g, Sugar: 3g, Sodium: 320 mg, Potassium: 450 mg, Cholesterol: 10 mg

BAKED FALAFEL WITH TZATZIKI SAUCE

PREPARATION TIME: 20 min
COOKING TIME: 25 min
MODE OF COOKING: Baking
SERVINGS: 4
INGREDIENTS:

- **Falafel:**
  - 1 can chickpeas, drained and rinsed
  - 1/4 cup fresh parsley, chopped
  - 1/4 cup fresh cilantro, chopped
  - 1/2 red onion, chopped
  - 2 cloves garlic, minced
  - 2 Tbsp flour
  - 1 tsp ground cumin
  - 1 tsp ground coriander
  - 1/2 tsp baking powder
  - Salt and pepper to taste
- **Tzatziki Sauce:**
  - 1 cup Greek yogurt
  - 1/2 cucumber, grated and drained
  - 1 Tbsp fresh lemon juice
  - 1 clove garlic, minced
  - 1 Tbsp fresh dill, chopped
  - Salt and pepper to taste

DIRECTIONS:

1. Preheat oven to 375°F (190°C). Line a baking sheet with parchment paper.
2. In a food processor, combine chickpeas, parsley, cilantro, red onion, garlic, flour, cumin, coriander, baking powder, salt, and pepper. Pulse until mixture is combined but still slightly chunky.
3. Form the mixture into small patties and place them on the prepared baking sheet.
4. Bake for 20-25 minutes, flipping halfway through, until golden brown and crispy.
5. In a small bowl, combine Greek yogurt, grated cucumber, lemon juice, garlic, dill, salt, and pepper to make the tzatziki sauce.
6. Serve the falafel with tzatziki sauce.

TIPS:

- Serve in pita bread with fresh vegetables for a delicious sandwich.
- Add a pinch of cayenne pepper to the falafel mixture for a spicy kick.

N.V.: Calories: 180, Fat: 8g, Carbs: 20g, Protein: 7g, Sugar: 3g, Sodium: 320 mg, Potassium: 300 mg, Cholesterol: 0 mg

SPINACH AND FETA STUFFED CHICKEN

PREPARATION TIME: 15 min
COOKING TIME: 25 min
MODE OF COOKING: Baking
SERVINGS: 4
INGREDIENTS:

- 4 boneless, skinless chicken breasts
- 1 cup fresh spinach, chopped
- 1/2 cup feta cheese, crumbled
- 1/4 cup sun-dried tomatoes, chopped
- 2 cloves garlic, minced
- 2 Tbsp olive oil
- Salt and pepper to taste

DIRECTIONS:

1. Preheat oven to 375°F (190°C). Line a baking sheet with parchment paper.
2. In a bowl, combine spinach, feta cheese, sun-dried tomatoes, and garlic.
3. Cut a slit in each chicken breast to create a pocket.
4. Stuff each chicken breast with the spinach mixture and secure with toothpicks.
5. Brush the chicken breasts with olive oil and season with salt and pepper.
6. Place the chicken breasts on the prepared baking sheet.
7. Bake for 25 minutes, or until the chicken is cooked through.
8. Serve immediately.

TIPS:

- Serve with a side of roasted vegetables or a Greek salad.
- Add a squeeze of lemon juice before serving for extra flavor.

N.V.: Calories: 260, Fat: 12g, Carbs: 2g, Protein: 34g, Sugar: 1g, Sodium: 350 mg, Potassium: 600 mg, Cholesterol: 100 mg

EGGPLANT PARMESAN

PREPARATION TIME: 20 min
COOKING TIME: 40 min
MODE OF COOKING: Baking
SERVINGS: 4
INGREDIENTS:

- 2 medium eggplants, sliced into rounds
- 2 cups marinara sauce
- 1 cup mozzarella cheese, shredded
- 1/2 cup Parmesan cheese, grated
- 1 cup whole wheat breadcrumbs
- 2 eggs, beaten
- 2 Tbsp olive oil
- 1 tsp dried oregano
- 1 tsp dried basil
- Salt and pepper to taste
- Fresh basil for garnish

DIRECTIONS:

1. Preheat oven to 375°F (190°C). Line a baking sheet with parchment paper.
2. Dip eggplant slices into beaten eggs, then coat with whole wheat breadcrumbs.
3. Arrange the eggplant slices on the prepared baking sheet and drizzle with olive oil.
4. Bake for 20 minutes, flipping halfway through, until golden brown.
5. In a baking dish, spread a thin layer of marinara sauce. Layer with baked eggplant slices, more marinara sauce, mozzarella cheese, and Parmesan cheese. Repeat layers.
6. Sprinkle dried oregano and basil over the top.
7. Bake for an additional 20 minutes, or until cheese is bubbly and golden.
8. Garnish with fresh basil before serving.

TIPS:

- Serve with a side of whole wheat pasta or a green salad.
- Use gluten-free breadcrumbs for a gluten-free option.

N.V.: Calories: 320, Fat: 16g, Carbs: 32g, Protein: 14g, Sugar: 8g, Sodium: 580 mg, Potassium: 700 mg, Cholesterol: 70 mg

•10.2 ASIAN INSPIRATIONS: GENTLE ON DIGESTION AND FULL OF FLAVOR.

GINGER CHICKEN STIR-FRY

PREPARATION TIME: 15 min
COOKING TIME: 15 min
MODE OF COOKING: Stir-frying
SERVINGS: 4
INGREDIENTS:

- 1 lb. chicken breast, thinly sliced
- 2 Tbsp soy sauce
- 1 Tbsp rice vinegar
- 1 Tbsp sesame oil
- 2 Tbsp fresh ginger, minced
- 2 cloves garlic, minced
- 1 red bell pepper, sliced
- 1 cup broccoli florets
- 1 cup snap peas
- 1/4 cup green onions, sliced
- 2 Tbsp olive oil
- 1 Tbsp honey
- 1 Tbsp cornstarch mixed with 2 Tbsp water
- Sesame seeds for garnish
- Cooked jasmine rice for serving

DIRECTIONS:

1. In a bowl, marinate chicken slices with soy sauce, rice vinegar, and sesame oil for 10 minutes.
2. Heat olive oil in a large skillet or wok over medium-high heat.
3. Add ginger and garlic, stir-fry for 1 minute until fragrant.
4. Add marinated chicken and cook until browned, about 5 minutes.
5. Add bell pepper, broccoli, and snap peas; stir-fry for another 3-4 minutes.
6. Stir in green onions and honey.
7. Add the cornstarch mixture and cook until the sauce thickens.
8. Garnish with sesame seeds and serve over jasmine rice.

TIPS:

- Use tofu instead of chicken for a vegetarian option.
- Add a splash of lime juice for extra freshness.

N.V.: Calories: 250, Fat: 10g, Carbs: 15g, Protein: 24g, Sugar: 7g, Sodium: 600 mg, Potassium: 550 mg, Cholesterol: 55 mg

MISO SOUP WITH TOFU AND SEAWEED

PREPARATION TIME: 10 min
COOKING TIME: 10 min
MODE OF COOKING: Boiling
SERVINGS: 4
INGREDIENTS:

- 4 cups water
- 1/4 cup miso paste
- 1 block tofu, cubed
- 1 cup seaweed, rehydrated
- 1/4 cup green onions, sliced
- 1/2 cup mushrooms, sliced
- 1 tsp sesame oil
- Soy sauce to taste

DIRECTIONS:

1. In a pot, bring water to a boil.
2. Add miso paste, stirring until dissolved.
3. Add tofu, seaweed, mushrooms, and green onions.
4. Simmer for 5-7 minutes until vegetables are tender.
5. Drizzle with sesame oil and soy sauce to taste before serving.

TIPS:

- Add a soft-boiled egg for extra protein.
- Use different types of mushrooms for added flavor.

N.V.: Calories: 90, Fat: 3g, Carbs: 8g, Protein: 6g, Sugar: 1g, Sodium: 450 mg, Potassium: 250 mg, Cholesterol: 0 mg

VEGETABLE SPRING ROLLS WITH PEANUT SAUCE

PREPARATION TIME: 20 min
COOKING TIME: N/A
MODE OF COOKING: No cooking
SERVINGS: 4
INGREDIENTS:

- **Spring Rolls:**
  - 8 rice paper wrappers
  - 1 cup carrots, julienned
  - 1 cup cucumbers, julienned
  - 1 cup red cabbage, shredded
  - 1 cup lettuce, shredded
  - 1/4 cup fresh mint leaves
  - 1/4 cup fresh cilantro leaves
- **Peanut Sauce:**
  - 1/4 cup peanut butter
  - 2 Tbsp soy sauce
  - 1 Tbsp hoisin sauce
  - 1 Tbsp rice vinegar
  - 1 tsp sesame oil
  - 1 Tbsp honey
  - 2-3 Tbsp water to thin

DIRECTIONS:

1. Dip each rice paper wrapper in warm water for 10-15 seconds to soften.
2. Lay the wrapper flat and place a small amount of each vegetable and herbs in the center.
3. Fold the sides over the filling, then roll tightly to form the spring roll.
4. In a bowl, whisk together peanut butter, soy sauce, hoisin sauce, rice vinegar, sesame oil, honey, and water until smooth.
5. Serve spring rolls with peanut sauce.

TIPS:

- Add cooked shrimp or chicken for added protein.
- Use a variety of herbs for a more complex flavor.

N.V.: Calories: 160, Fat: 8g, Carbs: 18g, Protein: 4g, Sugar: 6g, Sodium: 400 mg, Potassium: 250 mg, Cholesterol: 0 mg

TERIYAKI SALMON

PREPARATION TIME: 10 min
COOKING TIME: 15 min
MODE OF COOKING: Baking
SERVINGS: 4
INGREDIENTS:

- 4 salmon fillets
- 1/4 cup soy sauce
- 1/4 cup mirin
- 2 Tbsp honey
- 1 Tbsp rice vinegar
- 1 tsp fresh ginger, grated
- 1 clove garlic, minced
- 1 Tbsp sesame oil
- 1 Tbsp sesame seeds
- Green onions for garnish

DIRECTIONS:

1. Preheat oven to 375°F (190°C).

2. In a bowl, whisk together soy sauce, mirin, honey, rice vinegar, ginger, garlic, and sesame oil.
3. Place salmon fillets in a baking dish and pour the marinade over them.
4. Bake for 12-15 minutes until the salmon is cooked through and the sauce is caramelized.
5. Garnish with sesame seeds and green onions before serving.

TIPS:
- Serve with steamed rice and vegetables.
- Marinate the salmon for at least 30 minutes for more flavor.

N.V.: Calories: 300, Fat: 15g, Carbs: 12g, Protein: 28g, Sugar: 8g, Sodium: 700 mg, Potassium: 700 mg, Cholesterol: 70 mg

COCONUT CURRY CHICKEN

PREPARATION TIME: 15 min
COOKING TIME: 20 min
MODE OF COOKING: Simmering
SERVINGS: 4
INGREDIENTS:
- 1 lb. chicken breast, cubed
- 1 can (14 oz) coconut milk
- 2 Tbsp red curry paste
- 1 bell pepper, sliced
- 1 cup snap peas
- 1 cup carrots, sliced
- 1 onion, sliced
- 2 cloves garlic, minced
- 1 Tbsp fresh ginger, minced
- 2 Tbsp fish sauce
- 1 Tbsp brown sugar
- 1 Tbsp lime juice
- Fresh cilantro for garnish

DIRECTIONS:
1. In a large skillet, heat a bit of oil over medium heat. Add garlic, ginger, and onion; sauté until fragrant.
2. Add chicken cubes and cook until browned.
3. Stir in red curry paste and cook for 1 minute.
4. Pour in coconut milk and bring to a simmer.
5. Add bell pepper, snap peas, and carrots; cook until vegetables are tender, about 10 minutes.
6. Stir in fish sauce, brown sugar, and lime juice.
7. Garnish with fresh cilantro and serve with rice.

TIPS:
- Use tofu for a vegetarian version.
- Add a handful of spinach for extra greens.

N.V.: Calories: 320, Fat: 20g, Carbs: 14g, Protein: 24g, Sugar: 8g, Sodium: 800 mg, Potassium: 600 mg, Cholesterol: 70 mg

•**10.3 LATIN AMERICAN CLASSICS: SPICY YET SUITABLE FOR SENSITIVE STOMACHS.**

CHICKEN TACOS WITH AVOCADO LIME SAUCE

PREPARATION TIME: 20 min
COOKING TIME: 15 min
MODE OF COOKING: Grilling
SERVINGS: 4
INGREDIENTS:
- **Tacos:**
  - 1 lb. chicken breast, thinly sliced
  - 2 Tbsp olive oil
  - 1 tsp ground cumin
  - 1 tsp smoked paprika
  - 1/2 tsp garlic powder
  - 1/2 tsp onion powder
  - Salt and pepper to taste
  - 8 small corn tortillas
  - 1 cup shredded lettuce
  - 1/2 cup diced tomatoes
  - 1/4 cup chopped fresh cilantro
- **Avocado Lime Sauce:**
  - 1 ripe avocado
  - 2 Tbsp fresh lime juice
  - 1/4 cup Greek yogurt
  - 1 clove garlic, minced
  - Salt and pepper to taste

DIRECTIONS:
1. In a bowl, mix olive oil, cumin, smoked paprika, garlic powder, onion powder, salt, and pepper. Add chicken slices and toss to coat.

2. Preheat grill to medium-high heat. Grill chicken for 5-7 minutes per side until fully cooked.
3. While the chicken is grilling, prepare the avocado lime sauce. In a blender, combine avocado, lime juice, Greek yogurt, garlic, salt, and pepper. Blend until smooth.
4. Warm the corn tortillas on the grill or in a skillet.
5. Assemble the tacos: place grilled chicken on each tortilla, top with shredded lettuce, diced tomatoes, and cilantro. Drizzle with avocado lime sauce.

TIPS:
- Add a sprinkle of queso fresco for extra flavor.
- Use whole wheat tortillas for added fiber.

N.V.: Calories: 350, Fat: 18g, Carbs: 28g, Protein: 22g, Sugar: 3g, Sodium: 350 mg, Potassium: 700 mg, Cholesterol: 60 mg

---

BLACK BEAN AND SWEET POTATO ENCHILADAS

PREPARATION TIME: 25 min
COOKING TIME: 30 min
MODE OF COOKING: Baking
SERVINGS: 4
INGREDIENTS:
- **Filling:**
  - 1 large sweet potato, peeled and diced
  - 1 can black beans, drained and rinsed
  - 1/2 cup corn kernels
  - 1/2 cup diced red bell pepper
  - 1/2 cup diced onion
  - 2 cloves garlic, minced
  - 1 tsp ground cumin
  - 1/2 tsp chili powder
  - 2 Tbsp olive oil
  - Salt and pepper to taste
- **Enchiladas:**
  - 8 corn tortillas
  - 2 cups enchilada sauce
  - 1 cup shredded cheese (cheddar or Monterey Jack)
  - Fresh cilantro for garnish

DIRECTIONS:
1. Preheat oven to 375°F (190°C).
2. In a large skillet, heat olive oil over medium heat. Add sweet potato and cook until tender, about 10 minutes.
3. Add black beans, corn, red bell pepper, onion, garlic, cumin, chili powder, salt, and pepper. Cook for another 5 minutes until vegetables are tender.
4. Warm tortillas in the microwave or on the stovetop to make them pliable.
5. Spread 1/2 cup of enchilada sauce on the bottom of a baking dish.
6. Fill each tortilla with the sweet potato and black bean mixture, roll up, and place seam side down in the baking dish.
7. Pour the remaining enchilada sauce over the tortillas and sprinkle with shredded cheese.
8. Bake for 20-25 minutes until the cheese is melted and bubbly.
9. Garnish with fresh cilantro before serving.

TIPS:
- Serve with a side of Spanish rice.
- Add a dollop of sour cream on top for extra creaminess.

N.V.: Calories: 400, Fat: 16g, Carbs: 52g, Protein: 14g, Sugar: 8g, Sodium: 700 mg, Potassium: 900 mg, Cholesterol: 25 mg

---

PERUVIAN QUINOA SALAD

PREPARATION TIME: 15 min
COOKING TIME: 15 min
MODE OF COOKING: Boiling
SERVINGS: 4
INGREDIENTS:
- 1 cup quinoa, rinsed
- 2 cups vegetable broth
- 1 cup cherry tomatoes, halved
- 1/2 cup diced red bell pepper
- 1/2 cup diced cucumber
- 1/4 cup chopped red onion
- 1/4 cup fresh cilantro, chopped
- 1/4 cup fresh lime juice
- 2 Tbsp olive oil
- 1 clove garlic, minced
- Salt and pepper to taste

DIRECTIONS:

1. In a medium saucepan, bring vegetable broth to a boil. Add quinoa, reduce heat, cover, and simmer for 15 minutes, or until liquid is absorbed and quinoa is tender.
2. In a large bowl, combine cooked quinoa, cherry tomatoes, red bell pepper, cucumber, red onion, and cilantro.
3. In a small bowl, whisk together lime juice, olive oil, garlic, salt, and pepper.
4. Pour the dressing over the quinoa mixture and toss to combine.
5. Serve chilled or at room temperature.

TIPS:

- Add diced avocado for extra creaminess.
- Use red quinoa for a more colorful dish.

N.V.: Calories: 220, Fat: 9g, Carbs: 30g, Protein: 6g, Sugar: 4g, Sodium: 300 mg, Potassium: 550 mg, Cholesterol: 0 mg

BRAZILIAN FISH STEW (MOQUECA)

PREPARATION TIME: 15 min
COOKING TIME: 25 min
MODE OF COOKING: Simmering
SERVINGS: 4
INGREDIENTS:

- 1 lb. white fish fillets (such as cod or tilapia), cut into chunks
- 1 lime, juiced
- 2 Tbsp olive oil
- 1 onion, diced
- 1 red bell pepper, sliced
- 1 yellow bell pepper, sliced
- 2 cloves garlic, minced
- 1 can (14 oz) coconut milk
- 1 cup diced tomatoes
- 1/4 cup fresh cilantro, chopped
- 1 tsp paprika
- Salt and pepper to taste
- Fresh cilantro for garnish

DIRECTIONS:

1. In a bowl, marinate the fish with lime juice, salt, and pepper for 10 minutes.
2. In a large pot, heat olive oil over medium heat. Add onion, red bell pepper, yellow bell pepper, and garlic. Sauté until vegetables are tender.
3. Stir in coconut milk, diced tomatoes, cilantro, and paprika. Bring to a simmer.
4. Add the marinated fish to the pot and simmer for 10-15 minutes, or until the fish is cooked through.
5. Garnish with fresh cilantro before serving.

TIPS:

- Serve with white rice or crusty bread.
- Add a pinch of cayenne pepper for a bit of heat.

N.V.: Calories: 350, Fat: 20g, Carbs: 12g, Protein: 30g, Sugar: 6g, Sodium: 400 mg, Potassium: 850 mg, Cholesterol: 60 mg

MEXICAN STREET CORN SALAD

PREPARATION TIME: 10 min
COOKING TIME: 10 min
MODE OF COOKING: Grilling
SERVINGS: 4
INGREDIENTS:

- 4 ears of corn, husked
- 2 Tbsp olive oil
- 1/4 cup mayonnaise
- 1/4 cup Greek yogurt
- 1/4 cup crumbled cotija cheese
- 1 lime, juiced
- 1/2 tsp chili powder
- 1/4 cup chopped fresh cilantro
- Salt and pepper to taste

DIRECTIONS:

1. Preheat grill to medium-high heat. Brush the corn with olive oil.
2. Grill the corn, turning occasionally, until charred and cooked through, about 10 minutes.
3. Cut the corn kernels off the cob and place them in a large bowl.
4. In a small bowl, mix mayonnaise, Greek yogurt, lime juice, chili powder, salt, and pepper.
5. Add the dressing to the corn and toss to coat.
6. Stir in cotija cheese and cilantro.
7. Serve immediately.

TIPS:

- Use frozen corn if fresh is not available; simply sauté until charred.

- Add diced avocado for extra creaminess.

N.V.: Calories: 220, Fat: 14g, Carbs: 22g, Protein: 6g, Sugar: 6g, Sodium: 300 mg, Potassium: 350 mg, Cholesterol: 20 mg

Volume Measurements

US Measurement	Metric Measurement
1 tsp (tsp)	5 milliliters (ml)
1 tbsp (tbsp)	15 milliliters (ml)
1 fluid ounce (fl oz)	30 milliliters (ml)
1 Cup	240 milliliters (ml)
1 pint (2 Cs)	470 milliliters (ml)
1 quart (4 Cs)	0.95 liters (L)
1 gallon (16 Cs)	3.8 liters (L)

Weight Measurements

US Measurement	Metric Measurement
1 ounce (oz)	28 grams (g)
1 pound (lb)	450 grams (g)
1 pound (lb)	0.45 kilograms (kg)

Length Measurements

US Measurement	Metric Measurement
1 inch (in)	2.54 centimeters (cm)
1 foot (ft)	30.48 centimeters (cm)
1 foot (ft)	0.3048 meters (m)
1 yard (yd)	0.9144 meters (m)

Temperature Conversions

Fahrenheit (°F)	Celsius (°C)
32°F	0°C
212°F	100°C
Formula: (°F - 32) x 0.5556 = °C	Formula: (°C x 1.8) + 32 = °F

Oven Temperature Conversions

US Oven Term	Fahrenheit (°F)	Celsius (°C)
Very Slow	250°F	120°C
Slow	300-325°F	150-165°C
Moderate	350-375°F	175-190°C
Moderately Hot	400°F	200°C
Hot	425-450°F	220-230°C
Very Hot	475-500°F	245-260°C

CHAPTER 11: DINING OUT AND TRAVELING

Imagine you've just booked a trip, your suitcase packed with excitement and a tinge of worry. Travel and dining out, while thrilling, bring their own set of challenges when you're navigating life without a gallbladder. The blend of new cuisines and the unpredictability of meal timings might seem daunting, but with a few clever strategies, you can savor every meal without compromising your digestive health.

Traveling post-gallbladder removal doesn't mean you must forgo the joys of exploring local eateries or enjoying a meal at a bustling city café. The key lies in making informed choices that align with your dietary needs while still indulging in the cultural tapestry of your destination.

When dining out, the seemingly simple menu can appear like a maze of potential pitfalls. However, learning how to decode menu items and asking the right questions can turn it into a map guiding you to safe and delightful choices. Whether it's picking a restaurant that caters to dietary sensitivities or opting for dishes that are gentle on the system, these decisions empower you to maintain your health without missing out on flavorful experiences.

Moreover, traveling often tests your adaptability, but it also presents a unique opportunity to practice flexibility within your diet. Carrying a small stash of gallbladder-friendly snacks can be a lifesaver during long flights or layovers. Likewise, understanding how local food preparation techniques and ingredients affect your digestion will help you navigate new cuisines more comfortably.

Let's set the stage for a journey that's as fulfilling to your wanderlust as it is soothing to your stomach. By embracing these practices, you'll find that dining out and traveling can still be richly rewarding experiences. You'll return with not just memories of beautiful sights but also of joyous meals that kept you well-nourished and energized throughout your adventures. Remember, with the right preparation and mindset, every meal, no matter where in the world it's enjoyed, can be a step towards maintaining your digestive health and enhancing your travel experience.

•11.1 SELECTING GALLBLADDER-FRIENDLY RESTAURANT MEALS: HOW TO EAT OUT SAFELY.

Navigating the vibrancy of restaurant menus while keeping your digestive wellness in check may feel like balancing two contrasting ends of a spectrum. Yet, it is entirely possible to relish your dining experience without health compromises; it rests heavily on making informed, thoughtful choices. Here, we explore how to select gallbladder-friendly meals that promise both satisfaction and safety when dining out.

Embarking on a dining adventure begins long before you take your seat at a table. The art of selecting the right restaurant involves some initial research but pays dividends in ensuring a positive meal experience. Begin with browsing through online menus or calling the restaurant directly. Many dining establishments are now attuned to dietary restrictions and are often accommodating if they're aware ahead of time.

Once at the restaurant, open communication with your server is your gateway to a safe meal. It's beneficial to discuss your dietary needs plainly, emphasizing the necessity to avoid high-fat foods which are particularly taxing for those without a gallbladder. Most chefs appreciate knowing and understanding these requirements and can often suggest or modify dishes that cater to your needs. Understanding menu terminology is akin to learning a new dialect. Words like "grilled" or "steamed" are signals that the food is likely cooked in a manner suitable for your digestion. Conversely, descriptors such as "fried" or "creamy" are usually red flags, indicating dishes rich in fats and oils that can trigger discomfort. Embracing dishes centered around lean proteins, such as chicken, turkey, or fish, and pairing them with side dishes like steamed vegetables or salads dressed with a light vinaigrette, can be both satisfying and safe.

Portion control is another pivotal element. Restaurants often serve generous portions, which can be overwhelming for a digestive system that is adapting to life without a gallbladder. Consider ordering a half portion or sharing a meal with someone. This strategy not only keeps your digestion in check but also allows you to enjoy a broader range of flavors throughout your dining experience. An unanticipated challenge may arise with sauces and dressings, often hidden harbors of fats that can unsettle your digestive system. Asking for these to be served on the side allows you to control the amount you consume, and in some cases, it might be best to skip them altogether.

Eating slowly and mindfully plays a crucial role in digestive health. It's easy to rush through meals, especially in a social setting, but taking your time can help significantly. Eating slowly allows your digestive system to work without being overwhelmed, reducing potential post-meal discomforts like bloating or nausea.

And what about the delightful end to any meal—dessert? Opting for a fresh fruit plate or sorbet can satisfy the sweet craving without the heavy feeling associated with richer desserts. These lighter options provide a sweet finish without the digestive drama.

Let's not forget the cultural and local dietary practices while traveling. Each locale comes with its culinary identity, which can be both exciting and a bit intimidating from a dietary perspective. When traveling internationally, familiarize yourself with common local ingredients and cooking styles. This knowledge not only enriches your travel experience but also aids in making informed dining choices that align with your digestive needs.

Additionally, maintaining a small, well-curated list of "safe" snacks in your travel bag ensures you're never caught off guard when hunger strikes and suitable options are not immediately available. This foresight can be particularly beneficial during long layovers or when traveling through areas where finding gut-friendly food might pose a challenge.

Turning these practices into habits could transform your dining-out experiences drastically. It allows for embracing the joy of eating out and trying new foods while safeguarding your digestive health. Remember, every meal out is not just about eating; it's about enjoyment, social engagement, and embracing life's flavors without the side order of discomfort. With the right strategies, you can dine out confidently, making every meal a celebration of both flavor and well-being.

•11.2 SNACKS FOR TRAVEL: PORTABLE AND STOMACH-FRIENDLY.

There's a hidden magic in packing for a journey. Each item you choose to bring feels like it's part of a bigger narrative, a story about discovery and experience. When it comes to selecting food for travel, particularly for someone without a gallbladder, the priority shifts to balancing practicality with pleasure, ensuring each snack holds the power to nourish and satisfy without causing harm. The quest for the perfect travel snack is much like preparing for an expedition — both require foresight, preparation, and a keen understanding of the terrain, or in this case, your digestive health.

Navigational planning of your snacks is important, acting very much like setting waypoints on your journey. It starts with understanding what types of snacks work well, given your specific dietary needs. Post-cholecystectomy, this usually means focusing on options low in fat, easy to digest, yet filling and nutritious enough to sustain your energy levels while exploring new landscapes or enduring long transports.

Consider the virtues of whole, unprocessed foods. Fruits such as apples, bananas, and berries can be exceptional allies. They offer a rich source of vitamins and a quick, refreshing snack without burdening your stomach. Carrying a small sturdy container filled with these fruits can make them convenient and mess-free to eat on the go.

Vegetables, though less common as a travel snack, shouldn't be overlooked. Baby carrots, slices of bell pepper, or cherry tomatoes are not only crunchy and satisfying but also pack a bounty of nutrients without the high fat or calorie count that could upset your system. Paired with a small hummus pack, they can also provide enough fiber and protein to keep you satiated between meals.

Nuts and seeds, though higher in fat, can be included in moderation. Opt for those which are easier on the digestive system, like walnuts or pumpkin seeds, and avoid the salted or roasted varieties that could potentially lead to discomfort.

Let's not forget about hydration, an often-underestimated aspect of digestive health, particularly crucial for those without a gallbladder. Carrying a water bottle is imperative, but integrating herbal teas like ginger or peppermint can offer soothing properties and a pleasant change from plain water. These mild herbal teas can aid digestion and help keep nausea at bay, making your travel experience more comfortable.

Bringing along portable, non-perishable items can also be particularly useful. Oatmeal packets, for example, need just a touch of hot water to transform into a comforting meal. For a touch of sweetness, dried fruits like apricots or raisins can be a great choice; however, they should be consumed in moderation to manage sugar intake, which can sometimes exacerbate digestive issues.

Moreover, in today's world where many find themselves rushing from one terminal to another, having protein-rich bars can be a lifesaver. Opt for bars that are low in sugar and devoid of artificial sweeteners, focusing instead on those containing natural ingredients like date paste or almond butter.

The approach to packing snacks for travel should mirror how you might pack other essentials: lightweight, versatile, and prepared for unforeseen delays or changes. Each snack chosen should not only ease hunger but also align with your dietary restrictions, supporting your digestive health every step of the journey.

Now, while the snacks are packed and ready, another layer of navigation involves the ease of access. Keeping snacks within easy reach means you are less likely to find yourself desperate and grabbing whatever is available, which may not always align with your dietary needs. A well-placed, easily accessible snack pack in your carry-on can make all the difference in maintaining your dietary routine.

Though travel can be unpredictable, your approach to managing your health on the go should not be left to chance. By planning and packing with care, you create a buffer against the unforeseen, allowing you to enjoy the journey just as much as the destination itself. After all, travel is as much about the journey as it is about the destination, and maintaining your health makes the experience infinitely more enjoyable.

•11.3 TIPS FOR HEALTHY TRAVEL: HOW TO MAINTAIN YOUR DIET ON THE ROAD.

Traveling brings with it the allure of new experiences and the challenge of maintaining a consistent, digestive-friendly diet, particularly when you are without a gallbladder. The journey, much like life itself, requires adaptability and careful planning to ensure that your dietary needs are met even when you are miles away from the comforts of home. Here, we delve into tips that not only encourage maintaining your diet on the road but turn what could be a daunting prospect into a sequence of enjoyable experiences, each contributing to your overall well-being.

The cornerstone of healthy travel is preparation. Before you embark, spend time to research your destination. Understanding what food options will be available, locating grocery stores nearby, and checking if your accommodation offers a kitchenette all these factors play significant roles in keeping your diet on track. This foreknowledge reduces the uncertainty that often accompanies travel and sets a clear course for a smoother journey.

Another pivotal strategy is to communicate your needs clearly, whether you're booking your stay or ordering a meal. Don't hesitate to reach out to your hosts or servers about your specific dietary restrictions. Most places are accommodating and can provide valuable insights into local dining options that align with your dietary needs. This open communication not only helps you maintain your diet but may also introduce you to new, suitable local cuisines that you might not have otherwise discovered.

Packing for your dietary needs is just as important as packing clothes suitable for the weather. Always have on hand a selection of gallbladder-friendly snacks that travel well. This prepares you for any delays or limited food options during your travels. These snacks can be simple, like a mix of almonds and dried fruit kept handy in your travel bag, ensuring you have something to sustain you between meals.

Choosing accommodations wisely is another key aspect. Hotels with a mini-fridge or rental properties featuring a kitchenette can be invaluable. Having access to a place to store and possibly prepare some of your meals can make a significant difference. It allows you the freedom to control ingredients and portions, ensuring your meals are prepared in a way that suits your dietary restrictions.

Exercise moderation in all things, especially during the buffet-style meals that can be tempting on vacations. Smaller, more frequent meals are easier on your digestive system than large, infrequent ones. Opting for fresh, simply-prepared foods not only satisfies the palate but also supports your digestive health.

Hydration is crucial, particularly when travelling. However, be cautious with coffee, alcohol, and sugary drinks, which can disrupt your digestion system. Instead, opt for water or ginger tea, which aids digestion and can help prevent nausea often associated with travel.

In addition to what you eat and drink, consider the timing of your meals. Try to keep to your usual eating schedule as much as possible to maintain your body's rhythm. Regular meal times help regulate your digestive system, making it less likely that you'll experience discomfort.

While exploring, you might find yourself faced with a buffet of local delights, tempting you to try just a bit of everything. Remember, however, that the goal is not to restrict your experiences but to modify them in a way that respects your body's needs. Enjoy the local cuisine in moderation, mindful of how ingredients and preparation techniques might affect you. Grilled, baked, or steamed dishes typically are safer choices than fried or creamy ones.

Lastly, always carry a list of "safe foods" in the local language of the place you are visiting. This can be beneficial in avoiding misunderstandings and ensures that your dietary needs are clearly communicated.

In conclusion, maintaining your diet while on the road requires a balance of planning, communication, and discretion. By aligning your travel habits with these principles, you can enjoy every new experience without fear of digestive distress, turning each meal into an opportunity for pleasure and health. This approach not only supports your digestive health but also enhances your travel experience, allowing you to immerse fully in the moment without the underlying worry of a potential health setback.

CHAPTER 12: 45-DAY MEAL PLAN

Welcome to the core of your transformation - a carefully curated 45-day meal plan designed with your new lifestyle in mind. Striking the balance between nutrition and flavor, this plan isn't just a list of meals; it's a journey where each dish plays its part in harmonizing your digestive health and enhancing your overall well-being.

Imagine waking up each day, knowing exactly what delights await you on your plate—no guesswork, just a clear path towards a healthier you. This isn't about strict rules or the dull repetition of flavorless meals. Instead, it's about embracing a variety of foods that are as delicious as they are nourishing.

Now, I know adapting to life without a gallbladder presents its unique set of challenges. You've likely felt frustrated or overwhelmed by what to eat and what to avoid. This may have even caused some hesitancy to dine with joy. Let's brush those worries aside together. The coming pages are more than just a diet plan; they're a blueprint for eating well and living better.

Each week, we'll introduce meals that build upon one another, supporting your digestion and health without sacrificing taste. From invigorating breakfasts that kick-start your day to satisfying dinners that round it off, you'll find fresh, accessible recipes that align with your body's needs.

Alongside our day-to-day guide, we'll arm you with shopping lists and preparation tips that streamline your cooking process. More importantly, we'll delve into how to customize meals for your body's particular reactions, ensuring what lands on your table truly benefits you.

Let's start this path not just with the hope but with the certainty that within the next 45 days, you'll not only recalibrate your diet but rejuvenate your passion for food, armed with knowledge and flavored with joy.

•12.1 WEEKLY MEAL PLAN OVERVIEW: ORGANIZED EATING FOR DIGESTIVE HEALTH.

WEEK 1	breakfast	snack	lunch	snack	dinner
Monday	Tropical Sunrise Smoothie	Apple and Almond Butter Bites	Quinoa and Kale Salad	Greek Yogurt and Berry Parfait	Lemon Herb Grilled Chicken
Tuesday	Berry Blast Smoothie	Baked Zucchini Chips	Chickpea and Avocado Salad	Hummus and Veggie Sticks	Baked Salmon with Dill
Wednesday	Green Detox Smoothie	Cucumber and Hummus Bites	Mediterranean Lentil Salad	Banana and Almond Butter Roll-Ups	Quinoa-Stuffed Bell Peppers
Thursday	Creamy Avocado Smoothie	Sweet Potato Toasts with Avocado	Grilled Chicken and Arugula Salad	Roasted Chickpeas	Baked Cod with Lemon and Herbs
Friday	Protein Power Smoothie	Mini Caprese Skewers	Turkey and Avocado Wrap	Chia Pudding with Fresh Berries	One-Pot Chicken and Rice
Saturday	Quinoa and Berry Breakfast Bowl	Baked Apple Chips	Mediterranean Veggie Sandwich	Edamame with Sea Salt	Baked Salmon with Dill
Sunday	Savory Avocado and Egg Breakfast Bowl	Baked Carrot Fries	Chicken and Spinach Wrap	Avocado and Black Bean Dip with Veggie Sticks	One-Pot Pasta Primavera

WEEK 2	breakfast	snack	lunch	snack	dinner
Monday	Peanut Butter Banana Oatmeal Bowl	Coconut Date Balls	Beet and Goat Cheese Salad	Edamame with Sea Salt	Turkey Meatballs with Zucchini Noodles
Tuesday	Tropical Acai Breakfast Bowl	Baked Apple Chips	Tuna and Avocado Sandwich	Cucumber and Hummus Bites	Stuffed Bell Peppers with Quinoa and Black Beans
Wednesday	Sweet Potato and Spinach Breakfast Bowl	Avocado Toast with Cherry Tomatoes	Hummus and Veggie Wrap	Banana and Almond Butter Roll-Ups	Baked Salmon with Dill
Thursday	Classic Scrambled Eggs	Roasted Chickpeas	Ginger Carrot Soup	Apple and Almond Butter Bites	Baked Cod with Lemon and Herbs
Friday	Spinach and Feta Omelette	Chia Pudding with Fresh Berries	Chicken and Rice Soup	Greek Yogurt and Berry Parfait	One-Pot Chicken and Quinoa
Saturday	Veggie-Packed Egg Muffins	Baked Carrot Fries	Butternut Squash and Apple Soup	Mini Caprese Skewers	One-Pot Mediterranean Shrimp and Orzo
Sunday	Avocado Toast with Poached Eggs	Cucumber and Hummus Bites	Lentil and Spinach Soup	Hummus and Veggie Sticks	One-Pot Pasta Primavera
WEEK 3	breakfast	snack	lunch	snack	dinner
Monday	Spinach and Feta Omelette	Edamame with Sea Salt	Grilled Chicken and Arugula Salad	Greek Yogurt and Berry Parfait	Quinoa-Stuffed Bell Peppers
Tuesday	Green Detox Smoothie	Baked Zucchini Chips	Tuna and Avocado Sandwich	Roasted Chickpeas	One-Pot Pasta Primavera
Wednesday	Tropical Sunrise Smoothie	Avocado Toast with Cherry Tomatoes	Mediterranean Lentil Salad	Hummus and Veggie Sticks	Baked Cod with Lemon and Herbs
Thursday	Peanut Butter Banana Oatmeal Bowl	Mini Caprese Skewers	Quinoa and Kale Salad	Apple and Almond Butter Bites	One-Pot Chicken and Rice
Friday	Berry Blast Smoothie	Cucumber and Hummus Bites	Beet and Goat Cheese Salad	Baked Carrot Fries	Lemon Herb Grilled Chicken
Saturday	Savory Avocado and Egg Breakfast Bowl	Baked Apple Chips	Chicken and Spinach Wrap	Banana and Almond Butter Roll-Ups	Baked Salmon with Dill
Sunday	Protein Power Smoothie	Sweet Potato Toasts with Avocado	Mediterranean Veggie Sandwich	Chia Pudding with Fresh Berries	One-Pot Mediterranean Shrimp and Orzo

WEEK 4	breakfast	snack	lunch	snack	dinner
Monday	Avocado Toast with Poached Eggs	Coconut Date Balls	Ginger Carrot Soup	Roasted Chickpeas	Stuffed Bell Peppers with Quinoa and Black Beans
Tuesday	Creamy Avocado Smoothie	Baked Zucchini Chips	Chicken and Rice Soup	Apple and Almond Butter Bites	Turkey Meatballs with Zucchini Noodles
Wednesday	Tropical Acai Breakfast Bowl	Cucumber and Hummus Bites	Butternut Squash and Apple Soup	Hummus and Veggie Sticks	Baked Salmon with Dill
Thursday	Classic Scrambled Eggs	Baked Carrot Fries	Lentil and Spinach Soup	Greek Yogurt and Berry Parfait	Baked Cod with Lemon and Herbs
Friday	Sweet Potato and Spinach Breakfast Bowl	Mini Caprese Skewers	Mediterranean Veggie Sandwich	Edamame with Sea Salt	One-Pot Pasta Primavera
Saturday	Veggie-Packed Egg Muffins	Baked Apple Chips	Chicken and Spinach Wrap	Banana and Almond Butter Roll-Ups	Lemon Herb Grilled Chicken
Sunday	Quinoa and Berry Breakfast Bowl	Sweet Potato Toasts with Avocado	Mediterranean Lentil Salad	Chia Pudding with Fresh Berries	One-Pot Mediterranean Shrimp and Orzo

WEEK 5	breakfast	snack	lunch	snack	dinner
Monday	Protein Power Smoothie	Edamame with Sea Salt	Quinoa and Kale Salad	Greek Yogurt and Berry Parfait	Quinoa-Stuffed Bell Peppers
Tuesday	Berry Blast Smoothie	Baked Zucchini Chips	Tuna and Avocado Sandwich	Roasted Chickpeas	Lemon Herb Grilled Chicken
Wednesday	Tropical Sunrise Smoothie	Avocado Toast with Cherry Tomatoes	Mediterranean Lentil Salad	Hummus and Veggie Sticks	One-Pot Pasta Primavera
Thursday	Peanut Butter Banana Oatmeal Bowl	Mini Caprese Skewers	Beet and Goat Cheese Salad	Apple and Almond Butter Bites	One-Pot Chicken and Rice
Friday	Savory Avocado and Egg Breakfast Bowl	Cucumber and Hummus Bites	Butternut Squash and Apple Soup	Baked Carrot Fries	Baked Cod with Lemon and Herbs
Saturday	Creamy Avocado Smoothie	Baked Apple Chips	Chicken and Spinach Wrap	Banana and Almond Butter Roll-Ups	Baked Salmon with Dill
Sunday	Classic Scrambled Eggs	Sweet Potato Toasts with Avocado	Lentil and Spinach Soup	Chia Pudding with Fresh Berries	One-Pot Mediterranean Shrimp and Orzo

WEEK 6	breakfast	snack	lunch	snack	dinner
Monday	Quinoa and Berry Breakfast Bowl	Cucumber and Hummus Bites	Mediterranean Veggie Sandwich	Baked Carrot Fries	Baked Cod with Lemon and Herbs
Tuesday	Avocado Toast with Poached Eggs	Mini Caprese Skewers	Chicken and Spinach Wrap	Apple and Almond Butter Bites	Turkey Meatballs with Zucchini Noodles
Wednesday	Green Detox Smoothie	Sweet Potato Toasts with Avocado	Butternut Squash and Apple Soup	Greek Yogurt and Berry Parfait	One-Pot Chicken and Rice
Thursday	Tropical Acai Breakfast Bowl	Roasted Chickpeas	Tuna and Avocado Sandwich	Banana and Almond Butter Roll-Ups	Baked Salmon with Dill
Friday	Peanut Butter Banana Oatmeal Bowl	Edamame with Sea Salt	Lentil and Spinach Soup	Chia Pudding with Fresh Berries	One-Pot Pasta Primavera
Saturday	Savory Avocado and Egg Breakfast Bowl	Baked Zucchini Chips	Quinoa and Kale Salad	Hummus and Veggie Sticks	One-Pot Mediterranean Shrimp and Orzo
Sunday	Creamy Avocado Smoothie	Baked Apple Chips	Mediterranean Lentil Salad	Avocado Toast with Cherry Tomatoes	Lemon Herb Grilled Chicken
WEEK 7	breakfast	snack	lunch	snack	dinner
Monday	Spinach and Feta Omelette	Baked Apple Chips	Grilled Chicken and Arugula Salad	Roasted Chickpeas	One-Pot Mediterranean Shrimp and Orzo
Tuesday	Tropical Sunrise Smoothie	Sweet Potato Toasts with Avocado	Mediterranean Lentil Salad	Banana and Almond Butter Roll-Ups	Lemon Herb Grilled Chicken
Wednesday	Quinoa and Berry Breakfast Bowl	Mini Caprese Skewers	Chicken and Rice Soup	Greek Yogurt and Berry Parfait	One-Pot Chicken and Quinoa
Thursday	Berry Blast Smoothie	Cucumber and Hummus Bites	Butternut Squash and Apple Soup	Apple and Almond Butter Bites	Baked Cod with Lemon and Herbs
Friday	Avocado Toast with Poached Eggs	Baked Zucchini Chips	Tuna and Avocado Sandwich	Hummus and Veggie Sticks	Turkey Meatballs with Zucchini Noodles
Saturday	Green Detox Smoothie	Edamame with Sea Salt	Mediterranean Veggie Sandwich	Baked Carrot Fries	One-Pot Pasta Primavera
Sunday	Classic Scrambled Eggs	Coconut Date Balls	Quinoa and Kale Salad	Chia Pudding with Fresh Berries	Baked Salmon with Dill

Shopping List Week 1

Fruits:
- ☐ Banana
- ☐ Pineapple
- ☐ Orange juice
- ☐ Apple
- ☐ Kale
- ☐ Cherry tomatoes
- ☐ Cucumber
- ☐ Lemon
- ☐ Berries
- ☐ Mixed berries
- ☐ Green apple
- ☐ Lime
- ☐ Avocado
- ☐ Lettuce

Vegetables:
- ☐ Zucchini
- ☐ Red onion
- ☐ Spinach
- ☐ Bell pepper
- ☐ Carrot
- ☐ Celery
- ☐ Parsley
- ☐ Sweet potato
- ☐ Basil

Proteins:
- ☐ Chicken breast
- ☐ Chickpeas
- ☐ Salmon
- ☐ Feta cheese
- ☐ Cod
- ☐ Protein powder
- ☐ Turkey
- ☐ Chicken thighs
- ☐ Mozzarella balls

Grains and Legumes:
- ☐ Quinoa
- ☐ Lentils
- ☐ Whole wheat tortilla
- ☐ Black beans
- ☐ Rice

Dairy:
- ☐ Greek yogurt
- ☐ Almond milk
- ☐ Hummus

Others:
- ☐ Coconut water
- ☐ Almond butter
- ☐ Olive oil
- ☐ Honey
- ☐ Granola
- ☐ Garlic
- ☐ Thyme
- ☐ Paprika
- ☐ Parmesan
- ☐ Balsamic glaze
- ☐ Chia seeds
- ☐ Chicken broth
- ☐ Water
- ☐ Lemon juice
- ☐ Cheese

Shopping List Week 2

Fruits:
- ☐ Banana
- ☐ Berries
- ☐ Apple
- ☐ Cucumber
- ☐ Avocado
- ☐ Cherry tomatoes
- ☐ Lemon
- ☐ Dates
- ☐ Acai

Vegetables:
- ☐ Zucchini
- ☐ Beets
- ☐ Carrots
- ☐ Bell peppers
- ☐ Sweet potato
- ☐ Spinach
- ☐ Arugula
- ☐ Lettuce
- ☐ Celery

Proteins:
- ☐ Ground turkey
- ☐ Salmon
- ☐ Tuna

- [ ] Chickpeas
- [ ] Cod
- [ ] Chicken breast
- [ ] Chicken thighs
- [ ] Eggs
- [ ] Feta cheese
- [ ] Goat cheese

Grains and Legumes:
- [ ] Quinoa
- [ ] Black beans
- [ ] Whole grain bread

- [ ] Oats
- [ ] Whole wheat wrap
- [ ] Breadcrumbs
- [ ] Rice
- [ ] Chia seeds

Dairy:
- [ ] Greek yogurt
- [ ] Almond milk
- [ ] Milk
- [ ] Butter

Others:
- [ ] Sea salt

- [ ] Olive oil
- [ ] Paprika
- [ ] Honey
- [ ] Granola
- [ ] Walnuts
- [ ] Parmesan
- [ ] Vegetable broth
- [ ] Chicken broth
- [ ] Cinnamon
- [ ] Peanut butter

SHOPPING LIST WEEK 3

Fruits:
- [ ] Banana
- [ ] Pineapple
- [ ] Orange juice
- [ ] Apple
- [ ] Berries
- [ ] Mixed berries
- [ ] Green apple
- [ ] Lemon
- [ ] Cherry tomatoes
- [ ] Cucumber
- [ ] Avocado

Vegetables:
- [ ] Kale
- [ ] Spinach
- [ ] Zucchini
- [ ] Bell pepper
- [ ] Carrot
- [ ] Celery

- [ ] Parsley
- [ ] Arugula
- [ ] Beets
- [ ] Tomato

Proteins:
- [ ] Chicken breast
- [ ] Chickpeas
- [ ] Cod
- [ ] Chicken thighs
- [ ] Eggs
- [ ] Feta cheese
- [ ] Goat cheese
- [ ] Tuna
- [ ] Mozzarella balls
- [ ] Parmesan

Grains and Legumes:
- [ ] Quinoa
- [ ] Lentils
- [ ] Black beans

- [ ] Whole grain bread
- [ ] Oats
- [ ] Rice
- [ ] Pasta
- [ ] Corn
- [ ] Almond milk
- [ ] Hummus

Dairy:
- [ ] Greek yogurt
- [ ] Almond milk
- [ ] Milk

Others:
- [ ] Sea salt
- [ ] Olive oil
- [ ] Paprika
- [ ] Honey
- [ ] Granola
- [ ] Walnuts
- [ ] Parmesan

- ☐ Vegetable broth
- ☐ Chicken broth
- ☐ Cinnamon
- ☐ Peanut butter
- ☐ Balsamic glaze
- ☐ Garlic
- ☐ Thyme
- ☐ Coconut water

SHOPPING LIST WEEK 4

Fruits:
- ☐ Banana
- ☐ Berries
- ☐ Apple
- ☐ Lemon
- ☐ Lime
- ☐ Avocado
- ☐ Pineapple
- ☐ Mixed berries
- ☐ Mango
- ☐ Cherry tomatoes

Vegetables:
- ☐ Spinach
- ☐ Kale
- ☐ Zucchini
- ☐ Bell pepper
- ☐ Carrot
- ☐ Cucumber
- ☐ Sweet potato
- ☐ Broccoli
- ☐ Cauliflower
- ☐ Asparagus
- ☐ Arugula

Proteins:
- ☐ Chicken breast
- ☐ Chickpeas
- ☐ Salmon
- ☐ Eggs
- ☐ Greek yogurt
- ☐ Tofu
- ☐ Black beans
- ☐ Lentils
- ☐ Turkey
- ☐ Shrimp

Grains and Legumes:
- ☐ Quinoa
- ☐ Oats
- ☐ Brown rice
- ☐ Whole grain bread
- ☐ Whole wheat tortilla
- ☐ Chickpea flour
- ☐ Almond flour
- ☐ Chia seeds
- ☐ Hemp seeds

Dairy:
- ☐ Almond milk

- ☐ Feta cheese
- ☐ Cottage cheese
- ☐ Cheddar cheese

Others:
- ☐ Olive oil
- ☐ Honey
- ☐ Almond butter
- ☐ Peanut butter
- ☐ Walnuts
- ☐ Cashews
- ☐ Sesame seeds
- ☐ Soy sauce
- ☐ Tahini
- ☐ Garlic
- ☐ Ginger
- ☐ Turmeric
- ☐ Cinnamon
- ☐ Paprika
- ☐ Cumin
- ☐ Black pepper
- ☐ Salt
- ☐ Coconut milk

Fruits:
- ☐ Banana
- ☐ Apple
- ☐ Mixed berries
- ☐ Avocado
- ☐ Lemon
- ☐ Orange
- ☐ Mango
- ☐ Blueberries
- ☐ Strawberries
- ☐ Grapes
- ☐ Pineapple

Vegetables:
- ☐ Spinach
- ☐ Kale
- ☐ Bell pepper
- ☐ Carrot
- ☐ Cucumber
- ☐ Zucchini
- ☐ Sweet potato
- ☐ Broccoli
- ☐ Cauliflower
- ☐ Tomato
- ☐ Lettuce
- ☐ Arugula

- ☐ Red onion

Proteins:
- ☐ Chicken breast
- ☐ Salmon
- ☐ Eggs
- ☐ Greek yogurt
- ☐ Chickpeas
- ☐ Black beans
- ☐ Turkey
- ☐ Tofu
- ☐ Lentils
- ☐ Tuna
- ☐ Shrimp

Grains and Legumes:
- ☐ Quinoa
- ☐ Brown rice
- ☐ Whole grain bread
- ☐ Oats
- ☐ Whole wheat tortilla
- ☐ Almond flour
- ☐ Chia seeds
- ☐ Hemp seeds

Dairy:
- ☐ Almond milk
- ☐ Feta cheese

- ☐ Cottage cheese
- ☐ Cheddar cheese

Others:
- ☐ Olive oil
- ☐ Honey
- ☐ Almond butter
- ☐ Peanut butter
- ☐ Walnuts
- ☐ Cashews
- ☐ Sesame seeds
- ☐ Soy sauce
- ☐ Tahini
- ☐ Garlic
- ☐ Ginger
- ☐ Turmeric
- ☐ Cinnamon
- ☐ Paprika
- ☐ Cumin
- ☐ Black pepper
- ☐ Salt
- ☐ Coconut milk
- ☐ Vegetable broth
- ☐ Chicken broth
- ☐ Balsamic vinegar

Fruits:
- ☐ Banana
- ☐ Apple
- ☐ Mixed berries
- ☐ Avocado
- ☐ Lemon
- ☐ Orange
- ☐ Pineapple
- ☐ Blueberries
- ☐ Strawberries
- ☐ Grapes
- ☐ Mango

Vegetables:
- ☐ Spinach
- ☐ Kale
- ☐ Bell pepper
- ☐ Carrot
- ☐ Cucumber
- ☐ Zucchini
- ☐ Sweet potato
- ☐ Broccoli
- ☐ Cauliflower
- ☐ Tomato
- ☐ Lettuce
- ☐ Arugula

- ☐ Red onion
- ☐ Garlic
- ☐ Ginger

Proteins:
- ☐ Chicken breast
- ☐ Salmon
- ☐ Eggs
- ☐ Greek yogurt
- ☐ Chickpeas
- ☐ Black beans
- ☐ Turkey
- ☐ Tofu
- ☐ Lentils
- ☐ Tuna
- ☐ Shrimp

Grains and Legumes:
- ☐ Quinoa
- ☐ Brown rice
- ☐ Whole grain bread
- ☐ Oats
- ☐ Whole wheat tortilla
- ☐ Almond flour
- ☐ Chia seeds
- ☐ Hemp seeds

Dairy:
- ☐ Almond milk
- ☐ Feta cheese
- ☐ Cottage cheese
- ☐ Cheddar cheese

Others:
- ☐ Olive oil
- ☐ Honey
- ☐ Almond butter
- ☐ Peanut butter
- ☐ Walnuts
- ☐ Cashews
- ☐ Sesame seeds
- ☐ Soy sauce
- ☐ Tahini
- ☐ Turmeric
- ☐ Cinnamon
- ☐ Paprika
- ☐ Cumin
- ☐ Black pepper
- ☐ Salt
- ☐ Coconut milk
- ☐ Vegetable broth
- ☐ Chicken broth
- ☐ Balsamic vinegar

Fruits:
- ☐ Banana
- ☐ Apple
- ☐ Mixed berries
- ☐ Avocado
- ☐ Lemon
- ☐ Orange
- ☐ Pineapple
- ☐ Blueberries
- ☐ Strawberries
- ☐ Grapes
- ☐ Mango
- ☐ Pear

Vegetables:
- ☐ Spinach
- ☐ Kale
- ☐ Bell pepper
- ☐ Carrot
- ☐ Cucumber
- ☐ Zucchini
- ☐ Sweet potato
- ☐ Broccoli
- ☐ Cauliflower
- ☐ Tomato
- ☐ Lettuce
- ☐ Arugula
- ☐ Red onion
- ☐ Garlic
- ☐ Ginger
- ☐ Asparagus

Proteins:
- ☐ Chicken breast
- ☐ Salmon
- ☐ Eggs
- ☐ Greek yogurt
- ☐ Chickpeas
- ☐ Black beans
- ☐ Turkey
- ☐ Tofu
- ☐ Lentils
- ☐ Tuna
- ☐ Shrimp

Grains and Legumes:
- ☐ Quinoa
- ☐ Brown rice
- ☐ Whole grain bread
- ☐ Oats
- ☐ Whole wheat tortilla
- ☐ Almond flour
- ☐ Chia seeds
- ☐ Hemp seeds

Dairy:
- ☐ Almond milk
- ☐ Feta cheese
- ☐ Cottage cheese
- ☐ Cheddar cheese

Others:
- ☐ Olive oil
- ☐ Honey
- ☐ Almond butter
- ☐ Peanut butter
- ☐ Walnuts
- ☐ Cashews
- ☐ Sesame seeds
- ☐ Soy sauce
- ☐ Tahini
- ☐ Turmeric
- ☐ Cinnamon
- ☐ Paprika
- ☐ Cumin
- ☐ Black pepper
- ☐ Salt
- ☐ Coconut milk
- ☐ Vegetable broth
- ☐ Chicken broth
- ☐ Balsamic vinegar

Navigating the grocery store aisles can be both an adventure and a challenge, especially when adapting to a gallbladder-friendly diet. The key to success lies not only in knowing what to buy but also in understanding how to streamline the process so it enhances your lifestyle rather than complicates it. Here, we delve into practical tips and gentle guidance to make your shopping experience as rewarding and stress-free as cooking the meals themselves.

Starting with a well-planned shopping list can transform your trip from a tedious chore into a triumphant quest for health. Picture this: you enter the store, armed with a list that champions your dietary needs, directs your steps, and anchors your budget. This isn't just a list; it's your personal roadmap to nutritional success.

Embarking on Your Shopping Journey

Imagine navigating the grocery store with a clear focus. Your list is divided into sections corresponding to the store's layout, featuring fresh produce, proteins, dairy alternatives, and staples. This isn't by accident—it's a strategy to keep your cart filled with whole, unprocessed items that are the cornerstone of your new diet.

When it comes to fruits and vegetables, aim for variety and color, packing your cart with vibrant greens, deep reds, and sunny yellows. These are not only visually pleasing but packed with the vitamins and minerals essential to supporting your digestion and overall health.

Proteins: Lean but Mighty

Choosing proteins wisely is crucial; opt for lean cuts of meat, and incorporate plant-based proteins like lentils and chickpeas, which are kind to your digestion and add interesting textures to your meals. Fish, particularly rich in omega-3 fatty acids, should also feature prominently on your list, supporting your heart without overwhelming your digestive system.

Grains and Dairy Alternatives: Foundations of Flavor

Whole grains like quinoa, brown rice, and oats offer the dual benefits of fiber and comfort, integral to maintaining smooth digestion. Meanwhile, dairy alternatives such as almond milk or coconut yogurt provide the creamy textures you crave without the digestive downside, broadening the scope of your culinary endeavors.

The Art of Preparation

With your shopping complete, the next step is preparation. This phase is as much about mental preparation as it is about food. Approach your kitchen sessions with a plan that outlines not just what you're going to cook but also how you can make the process as efficient as possible.

Batch Cooking: A Time-Saving Miracle

Consider the art of batch cooking: preparing larger quantities of staples like rice or vegetables at the beginning of the week. This method not only saves time but also ensures that you have healthy components ready to transform into quick, delicious meals on busier days.

Smart Storage Solutions

Effective storage is another key aspect. Invest in quality storage containers that keep your food fresh and organize your ingredients in clear, accessible ways. Labeling items with cooking instructions and dates can make decision-making simpler throughout the week, reducing food waste and keeping your diet on track.

Timing Is Everything

When it comes to meal prep, timing can make or break your routine. Develop a rhythm by allocating specific times for prep. Perhaps Sunday afternoon is your chopping and roasting time, while Wednesday night is for assembling dishes that utilize those prepped ingredients. By setting these routines, you anchor your meal prep within your weekly schedule, making it a familiar and manageable ritual.

Embracing Flexibility

However, it's important to remain flexible. Life can be unpredictable, and dietary needs may shift. Listen to your body and adjust your meal plan as needed. Maybe one week you find that certain foods aren't settling well, or you're craving more of another. This adjustment is not a setback but an integral part of tailoring a diet that suits your unique post-gallbladder removal life.

Reflecting on this overview, remember that your shopping list and prep routines are more than just tasks—they are integral parts of a holistic approach to health. They empower you to take control, minimize stress, and maximize enjoyment of your meals. Each carefully planned and prepared meal is a step towards revitalizing your digestive health and reclaiming the joy of eating. Approach each step as part of a greater journey towards wellness. With each item you check off your list and every meal you prep in advance, you are building a foundation for a healthier, more joyful way of life.

•12.3 CUSTOMIZING YOUR DIETARY PLAN: ADAPTING TO PERSONAL NEEDS AND PREFERENCES.

No two journeys through life—or through post-gallbladder removal—are precisely the same. Each of us, unique in our tastes and physiological reactions, requires somewhat personalized approaches to managing our diet. This section delves into the dynamic and creative process of tailoring your 45-day meal plan to fit not just the common roadmap of nutritional needs but your personal preferences, quirks sensitivities, and lifestyle.

Embracing Individuality in Your Diet

Customizing your diet begins with a profound and empathetic understanding of your own body. Listening to how you react to different foods is more than just noting what works and what doesn't; it involves understanding your palate, your body's signals, and how various ingredients impact your overall well-being. This attunement can guide you to tweak and transform the meal plans into something uniquely suited to your digestive landscape.

The Feedback Loop

Think of the first few weeks of any new dietary plan as a conversation between you and your body. Introduce foods slowly, and gauge your body's reactions. This feedback, whether it's a sense of energization or discomfort, helps in fine-tuning your meal plan. Documenting how different foods make you feel can provide invaluable insights that go beyond generic dietary recommendations. This diary becomes a powerful tool, serving as your guide to molding a diet plan that truly resonates with your health needs.

Adjusting Macro and Micro-nutrients

The balance of macronutrients—proteins, fats, and carbohydrates—plays a crucial role in digestion, especially without a gallbladder. You might find that a higher intake of lean proteins and a moderate amount of healthy fats work best, or perhaps, your system prefers a rich variety of fibrous carbohydrates. Alongside macronutrients, tweaking micronutrients like vitamins, minerals, and enzymes based on how your body responds can further enhance digestive ease and energy levels.

Portion and Frequency Adjustments

Your eating schedule and portion sizes are just as pivotal to tailor. Smaller, more frequent meals can alleviate the burden on your digestive system, maintaining a steadier flow of bile from the liver into the intestines. Experiment with the size and frequency of meals to find what helps maintain your energy levels without causing bloating or discomfort.

Flavor Profiling

Customizing doesn't stop with the ingredients or portions; it extends into the realms of flavors and seasonings. The right herbs and spices can not only enhance taste but can serve to support digestion and mitigate inflammation. If a recipe calls for a spice that doesn't agree with you or isn't to your liking, finding a substitute that fulfills the same role without the discomfort is a creative pivot toward meal satisfaction.

Managing Food Intolerances

Post-gallbladder removal might also change how your body handles certain foods, potentially developing temporary or prolonged sensitivities. Identifying these and finding acceptable alternatives that provide similar nutritional benefits allows you to maintain a diverse and enjoyable diet. This adaptability ensures you don't feel restricted, keeping your meals enjoyable and healthful.

Integration into Lifestyle

Adapting your meal plan also means considering the rhythm of your daily life. Your meals should fit seamlessly into your schedule, providing convenience without compromising on health. This might mean preparing breakfasts that are quick to assemble on busy mornings or having go-to snacks ready for sudden midday hunger pangs.

Family and Social Considerations

Furthermore, your dietary needs should not alienate you from family meals or social gatherings. Customizing recipes to be both gallbladder-friendly and appealing to others ensures you can enjoy the warmth of shared meals without feeling sidelined. For instance, a common dish like a stew can be easily adapted using lean meats and low-fat techniques to suit your needs while remaining a family favorite.

Long-Term Adjustments

Finally, remember that your dietary needs may evolve. What works in the initial weeks might require adjustments as your body heals and adapts. This ongoing customization isn't just about maintaining comfort but about optimizing your diet for a vibrant, active life.

Through this personalized approach, your diet becomes more than a mere assembly of foods; it transforms into a supportive, enjoyable, and living plan that adjusts as you progress through your post-gallbladder removal journey. The goal is clear: to enable a lifestyle where managing your diet becomes second nature, allowing you to thrive in every other aspect of life. Customizing your meal plan isn't just about catering to personal tastes—it's about empowering you to create a flexible, responsive, and joyful eating experience.

CHAPTER 13: LONG-TERM SUCCESS AND WELLBEING

As you turn the pages and explore the depths of this dietary journey after losing your gallbladder, reaching Chapter 13 marks a significant milestone. It's here that we pause to reflect, not just on the concrete strategies and meal plans we've mastered, but on the deeper rhythm of well-being that integrates these elements into a symphony of sustained health.

Imagine standing at the intersection of diligent planning and spontaneous living, where you've learned to embrace both the structured dietary regime and the unforeseen circumstances that test your adaptability. It's at this juncture that your commitment transforms from a measured, temporary effort into a seamless part of your everyday life.

Thinking back to the early days post-surgery, your concerns might have centered on immediate relief and avoidance of discomfort, navigating through a plethora of dos and don'ts. However, over time, and through the pages of this guide, an evolution occurs—a gradual shift from reactive living to proactive thriving. This transformation is not just about avoiding certain foods or including others but understanding and feeling the pulse of a life well-nourished and well-celebrated despite the absence of your gallbladder.

The road to long-term success is paved with more than good intentions and dietary lists; it requires a mental shift, a kind of dietary mindfulness that attunes you to the needs and responses of your body and to the joy of feeding it well. Each recipe tried, each tip implemented serves as a building block in the robust foundation of your health.

Thus, as we delve into this final chapter, remember that this is not just an endpoint. It's a commencement—a celebration of the knowledge you've gained and the habits you've formed that will support your digestive wellness for years to come. Here, we'll consolidate your learning, reinforcing not just how to eat, but how to live—with vitality, with pleasure, and with a newfound respect for the body's remarkable ability to adapt and thrive.

•13.1 REFLECTING ON YOUR DIETARY CHANGES: UNDERSTANDING YOUR PROGRESS.

Embarking on a journey toward better health, especially after gallbladder removal, is akin to learning a new language. At first, there's a struggle to understand the basics — from identifying which foods to avoid to adopting a completely new dining routine. Now, as you reflect on your dietary changes, it's essential to gauge the distance traveled, to appreciate the shifts not just on your plate but in your mindset and overall health.

When you first stepped into this new culinary world, determined yet perhaps a bit overwhelmed, your kitchen seemed a strange, uncharted land where every meal required contemplation and each ingredient was scrutinized. Fast forward to today: you likely find yourself more in tune with this altered way of cooking and eating — more confident, innovative, and, importantly, more synchronized with your body's responses.

To fully embrace and understand this evolution, consider the initial hurdles you encountered. You may recall moments of frustration, perhaps during a family gathering or a meal out with friends, where your dietary restrictions felt more like burdens than steps toward better health. Reflect on these instances with compassion towards yourself. Acknowledge how you navigated those challenges, armed with increasing knowledge and an expanding toolkit of recipes and strategies that prioritize your well-being.

The Power of Adaptation

Adjusting your diet necessitates a combination of self-awareness and creativity. It wasn't merely about substituting non-compliant foods but reimagining meals that could both heal and satisfy. This journey likely nurtured a newfound patience for trial and error — discovering what meals could keep you nourished without triggering discomfort. You've morphed from following strict guidelines to becoming adept at tweaking recipes, crafting meals that are as pleasing to the palate as they are beneficial to your digestive system.

It is advantageous to periodically keep a food diary, not just as a record of what you eat but how you feel physically and emotionally after each meal. Such reflections can highlight patterns that may not be immediately obvious — like identifying specific ingredients that agree particularly well with your system or recognizing times of day when your energy levels peak and dip.

Celebrating the Victories

While managing dietary needs can be complex, each success deserves recognition. Whether it's mastering a new cooking technique or noticing fewer digestive upsets, these victories significantly contribute to your health journey. Celebrate the fact that meals have become more than sustenance; they are a tribute to your resilience and dedication.

One significant triumph is the transformation in your relationship with food. It's possible you've discovered how certain textures or flavors work in symphony to create dishes that support your digestive processes, where once they might have caused alarm. Reflecting on such accomplishments can be profoundly uplifting, a reminder of your ability to adapt and thrive.

Long-term Insights

Having adapted to this dietary shift, your understanding of nutrition likely deepened. You've become not just a follower of recipes but a scholar of ingredients, understanding their roles and impacts. This knowledge enriches your life beyond the confines of diet; it influences your choices at grocery stores, restaurants, and even in conversations with others about health.

Reflect on how this journey could guide others around you. Many find inspiration from watching someone tackle health challenges with grace and determination. Your experiences and the insights you've gained could serve as a beacon for others facing similar struggles, providing both practical advice and emotional support.

The Journey Ahead

Looking forward, your dietary journey is far from over. It will continue to evolve, just as your body and health needs will. Anticipate future adaptations with a sense of curiosity and confidence, knowing that you are equipped with the knowledge and skills to manage whatever comes your way. The integration of these dietary practices into your daily life is a profound testament to your dedication to health and well-being.

Take a moment to visualize where you might be a few years from now — perhaps introducing new, tantalizing dishes to your repertoire or sharing your story with those who are newly navigating life without a gallbladder. Envision a future where you continue to refine your dietary routine, not just to prevent discomfort but to proactively enhance your wellbeing.

The insights garnered through your reflective process underscore a simple truth: that the journey towards health, especially after such a significant physical change, is continuous. Each day presents new challenges and opportunities to cultivate well-being. With each passing meal and mastered recipe, you reaffirm your commitment to a vibrant, health-focused life. Celebrate where you are today and approach the future with anticipation and enthusiasm for the ongoing journey of health and discovery.

•13.2 STRATEGIES FOR SUSTAINED HEALTH: MAINTAINING DIGESTIVE WELLNESS.

In the continuous journey towards sustaining health after your gallbladder removal, consider how far you've traveled and the horizon that yet beckons. This enduring quest for wellbeing, especially in maintaining digestive wellness, is not merely about adherence to specific dietary guidelines. Instead, it encompasses a holistic approach that blends lifestyle choices with keen nutritional awareness, fostering a long-lasting vitality that transcends ordinary dieting.

Imagine your path to sustained health as weaving a tapestry, where each thread represents different aspects of your lifestyle——nutrition, exercise, mental health, and emotional well-being. Over time, these threads intertwine to form a resilient and beautiful whole, improving not only your digestive health but your overall quality of life.

Building a Flexible, Nutrient-Rich Diet

A key component in maintaining your digestive health lies in adopting a flexible approach to eating. It's about creating a diet that is responsive to your body's changing needs and the realities of daily life. Recognize that while certain foods should generally be minimized or avoided, such as overly fatty meats or high-fat dairy products, the real art lies in balancing these with a bounty of foods that nourish and heal.

Your diet should be rich in fiber, which aids in digestion and helps prevent constipation, a common issue post-gallbladder surgery. Include a variety of fruits, vegetables, whole grains, and legumes——each offering unique fibers, antioxidants, and other nutrients that contribute to gut health. But more than just being inclusive, be mindful of your body's responses to these foods; what works for one may not work for another. This awareness allows you to customize your diet continually, ensuring it meets your evolving health needs.

Emphasizing Regular Physical Activity

Physical activity is an equally important thread in your wellness tapestry. Not only does regular exercise help maintain a healthy weight, but it also stimulates normal bowel function. Think of movement as a massage for your digestive tract, enhancing motility and alleviating symptoms like bloating and gas.

Integrate activities you enjoy into your routine to ensure consistency. Whether it's brisk walking, cycling, swimming, or yoga, the best exercise is the one you look forward to performing regularly. It's less about intensity and more about regularity; even a daily 30-minute walk can make a significant difference in your digestive health and overall vitality.

Managing Stress Effectively

Often underestimated, stress plays a crucial role in digestive health. High stress levels can exacerbate gut symptoms and disturb the delicate balance of your digestive system. Cultivating effective stress management techniques is essential. Practices like mindfulness meditation, deep breathing exercises, and engaging in hobbies that relax you can profoundly affect your stress levels and, by extension, your gut health.

Develop a routine that includes moments of calm and mindfulness. These practices do more than soothe your mind; they create conditions under which your digestive system can operate optimally. By managing stress, you're not just caring for your mind but also nurturing your body.

Ensuring Regular Medical Check-ups

Regular consultations with healthcare professionals play a critical role in maintaining long-term health. These check-ups provide an opportunity to assess your condition, monitor the effectiveness of your dietary strategy, and make necessary adjustments. Your doctor can help you navigate the complex interactions between diet and health, offering insights tailored to your specific needs.

Do not underestimate the value of these professional relationships in your pursuit of wellness. They act as your guideposts, ensuring that your journey is supported by scientific understanding and specialized insights.

Educating Yourself Continuously

The landscape of health information is constantly evolving. Staying informed about the latest research and recommendations for managing life without a gallbladder is key to maintaining your health. Invest time in learning from reputable sources, participating in workshops, or joining support groups where experiences and knowledge are shared.

Your education is your empowerment; understanding the why behind the advice you follow enhances your commitment to these practices. This ongoing learning process not only keeps you informed but also motivated, reinforcing the importance of the dietary and lifestyle choices you make every day.

Nurturing Social Connections

Finally, the support of friends, family, and community is invaluable. Sharing meals, discussing your challenges and successes, and receiving encouragement can incredibly enhance your well-being. These social interactions are not just emotionally fulfilling; they can also offer practical support in maintaining your health routines.

Involve your loved into your wellness journey. Cooking together, sharing recipes, and even exploring new food-related experiences can make maintaining your health regimen more enjoyable and less isolating.

The journey towards sustained health, particularly in maintaining digestive wellness, is both challenging and rewarding. It requires attention to diet, exercise, stress management, regular medical oversight, continuous education, and the cultivation of supportive social networks. Each of these components intertwines to create a comprehensive approach to health that supports not only your digestive system but your entire well-being, paving the way for a fulfilling, vibrant life post-gallbladder removal.

•13.3 RESOURCES FOR ONGOING SUPPORT: CONTINUING YOUR HEALTH JOURNEY.

The journey to maintaining health, especially after a significant medical change such as gallbladder removal, is just like venturing through a vast, diverse landscape—it requires a reliable map and the support of fellow travelers. As you continue to navigate this transformative path, utilizing a variety of resources will safeguard your progress, ensuring that your steps towards digestive wellness are both informed and supported.

Harnessing the Power of Digital Platforms

In today's interconnected world, digital resources are invaluable for staying current on the latest in health and nutrition. Websites, mobile apps, and online forums not only provide access to the most recent research and advice but also connect you with a global community of individuals sharing similar experiences. Reliable health websites managed by medical professionals or reputed health organizations offer articles, podcasts, and videos that explain complex information in understandable terms.

Mobile apps designed for dietary management can be particularly helpful. They can help you track your meals, monitor symptoms, and even provide tips for dietary adjustments. Moreover, forums and online support groups offer emotional solidarity and practical advice, making the journey less isolating.

Leveraging Books and Publications

While the digital age offers immediacy and connectivity, books and publications remain priceless resources for in-depth understanding. They provide a structured approach to learning and are often peer-reviewed, ensuring the accuracy and reliability of the information. For anyone navigating the post-gallbladder removal landscape, books on digestive health, wellness, and nutrition offer insights and strategies that are both time-tested and innovative.

Medical journals and articles can also serve as excellent tools for those who wish to delve deeper into the scientific aspects of their condition. They present research findings and expert analyses that can enhance your understanding of how dietary choices impact digestive health.

Engaging with Healthcare Professionals

Ongoing support from healthcare professionals is crucial in adapting your dietary and lifestyle habits to your body's needs after gallbladder removal. Nutritionists, dietitians, and gastroenterologists can provide personalized advice based on the latest medical insights. Regular appointments allow for adjustments to your dietary plan as your digestive system adapts, ensuring that recommendations stay aligned with your health status.

Moreover, many healthcare providers offer workshops, seminars, and training sessions that can be incredibly beneficial. These sessions often address common concerns and provide a platform to ask questions and interact with experts directly.

Participating in Workshops and Seminars

Workshop and seminar participation can enhance your knowledge and skills, providing fresh perspectives on managing your health. These sessions often cover a range of topics, including meal planning, understanding and managing symptoms, and psychological coping strategies, which are essential for long-term dietary management.

Local community centers, hospitals, or wellness clinics frequently host such events, offering an opportunity to learn in a supportive group environment. Additionally, cooking classes can also be beneficial, providing hands-on experience with preparing foods that cater to your specific dietary needs.

Integrating Community and Support Networks

The value of a supportive community cannot be overstated. Engaging with local support groups or online communities focused on gallbladder health, digestion issues, or general wellness can provide moral support, encouragement, and shared experiences. These networks can be particularly helpful during challenging times, offering both understanding and motivation.

Local support groups often organize regular meetings where members can share their experiences, challenges, and successes. Participating in these meetings can enhance your sense of connection and belonging, reducing feelings of isolation and helping you stay committed to your health goals.

Staying Informed through Conferences and Health Expos

Health conferences and expos present opportunities to discover emerging therapies, cutting-edge nutritional research, and innovative products that can support digestive health. These events gather experts from diverse fields, offering lectures, panel discussions, and booths with educational materials and samples.

Attending such conferences enables you to stay at the forefront of medical and nutritional research, directly enhancing your capability to manage your health effectively. They also provide a unique opportunity to ask questions, gather resources, and even sample new products that are conducive to maintaining digestive wellness.

The varied landscape of resources available to you is rich with information and support. Digital platforms, books, consultations with health professionals, workshops, community support networks, and health conferences all play integral roles in supporting your ongoing health journey. By strategically utilizing these resources, you can maintain your path to sustained health, ensuring that each step forward is as informed and supported as possible. As you continue to traverse this path, remember that each resource is a tool at your disposal, ready to help you manage and thrive in your life post-gallbladder removal.

Made in the USA
Las Vegas, NV
06 April 2025

20602759R00059